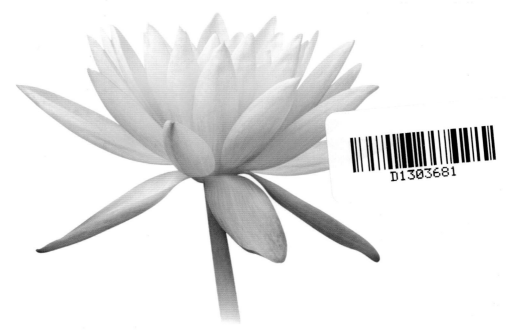

SLOW AGEING GUIDE TO

SKIN
REJUVENATION

LEARN • UNDERSTAND • SELECT • PROVEN TREATMENTS

First published 2016
Copyright 2016 Health Inform Pty Ltd©

Published by Health Inform Pty Ltd
PO Box 95
Ingleburn
NSW, 1890
Tel: +61 414517122
www.slowaging.org
content@slowaging.org

Authors: Kate Marie, Professor Merlin Thomas with Dr John Flynn
Publisher: Carolen Barripp
Printed in Singapore by 1010 Printing International

National Library of Australia
Cataloguing-in-Publication data:
Marie, Kate, 1962-
Slow Ageing Guide to Skin Rejuvenation
Kate Marie, Professor Merlin Thomas with Dr John Flynn
Includes index.
ISBN: 978-0-9806339-1-7

Disclaimer: Every effort has been made to ensure that the information in this book is as accurate as possible. The publisher, authors and contributors have taken every care in the preparation of this book, but do not warrant that the information it contains will be free from error or omissions, or that it will be suitable for the reader's purposes. The publisher, authors and contributors are not responsible for any adverse effects or consequences resulting from the use of any suggestions, interventions or opinions contained in this book. Nothing in this book should be interpreted as medical advice and the information in this book is not intended as a substitute for consulting with your doctor, skin practitioner or other health care provider. All matters relating to your health and skin should be discussed with a doctor or authorised practitioner.

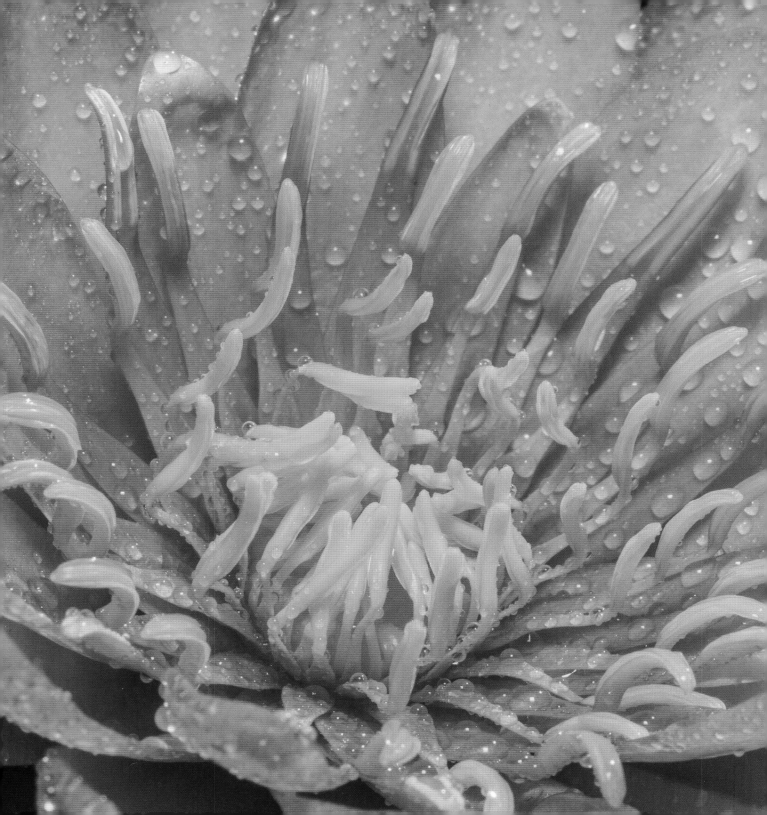

CONTENTS

TESTIMONIALS

There is much you can do to look after your skin, but it can become confusing and make you want to give up. This book gives you the information you need to make the right decisions about what is best for you and your skin.
Dr Joe Kosterich

Our skin is an outward reflection of our whole health and wellbeing. This book explores a holistic approach to skin health, is a wealth of information and it should be on everyone's bookshelf.
Dr Danielle Arabina

As a qualified nurse working in acute and aged care settings, I know how important it is that good skin integrity is maintained. Adopting robust health practices is the only way to do this, and this wonderful book makes it easy by showing you the way.
Kathleen Lanaghan

This book is a fantastic guide. It has provided me with all the information I need to help me make decisions about what I want to do – and what I didn't want to do – with my skin to help me look and feel amazing.
Sharon St Pierre

I like to be fully informed and not be a victim to the cosmetic industry. My skin care has to be sustainable for the long term and offer actual impact. This book has helped me understand how my skin works and then work out my own plan of action – just right for me. It has helped me put my best face forward!
Margo Field

As a 40-year-old male who has never paid attention to skin starting to hit a point where I should – this book is the best on the market.
Amit Vohra

AUTHORS

Kate Marie

Kate Marie has worked in the health industry for over 30 years. Starting out as a nurse, she has subsequently worked in sales, marketing, business development and digital strategy for a number of health and medical organisations, including the Royal Australian College of General Practitioners, GP Training Queensland and General Practice Registrars Australia. She founded two dotcoms in the heady days of the 1990s before the market crashed and caused a re-think on how to bring the 'e' into health. Kate is currently the director of business development at Content Doctor and CEO of Thrive, a start-up social enterprise. She is the founder of the Slow Ageing movement and a contributing author of the book *Fast Living Slow Ageing*. Kate's mission in life is to help women to better navigate the ageing process and embrace their fifties and beyond as a time to optimise personal health and wellbeing and to live a life of purpose and contribution.

Professor Merlin Christopher Thomas MD, PhD

Professor Thomas is both a physician and a scientist, working in Melbourne, Australia. His research primarily focuses on diabetes and its complications, and finding practical means for their control. But he has a broader interest in all aspects of preventive medicine and ageing. He has published over 270 articles in many of the worlds' leading medical journals, as well as several bestselling books including Understanding Type 2 Diabetes, and was a contributing author to *Fast Living Slow Ageing*. He is internationally recognised as a speaker, opinion-leader, teacher and medical storyteller.

Dr John Flynn MBBS, Dip RACOG, FRACGP, Dip.P.Derm, FACCS

Dr Flynn graduated from The University of Queensland Medical School in 1976. He has obtained a Dermatology qualification in the UK, is certified by the American Board of Laser Surgery, is a Fellow of the Australasian College of Cosmetic Surgery, for whom he is currently the Censor in Chief of the College and was formerly President. Dr Flynn specialises in facial cosmetic surgery and non-invasive facial rejuvenation techniques. He developed the SafFe Lift, a technique of minimally invasive facial rejuvenation that is popular in Australia, Southeast Asia and the USA. Dr Flynn is regularly invited to present at academic meetings in Australia and internationally. He has taught cosmetic surgeons, physicians, plastic surgeons, ophthalmologists, and dermatologists in Australia and overseas. He presents training courses in facial contouring using injectable fillers and is a contributing author to texts on cosmetic surgery. Dr Flynn consults for pharmaceutical companies on products and has assisted in development programs. He has conducted surveys of adverse events in cosmetic surgery and medicine to ascertain proper treatment strategies and the results of this work are now featured in product information and risk management profiles internationally.

CONTRIBUTORS

Dr Geoffrey Heber MBBS (UNSW), MBA (Syd)

Dr Heber is a Fellow of the Cosmetic Physicians College of Australia. He has been a principal of Heber Davis Cosmetic Medicine, founded in 1988 and one of the first few dedicated and largest cosmetic medical practices in Australia. In 1991 commenced distributing various international cosmetic brands in Australasia and in 1998 he founded the Australian skincare company Ultraceuticals which is distributed internationally.

Ann-Mary Hromek RN, ND, FACNEM(hon), FINMA, MATMS

Ann-Mary completed her General Nursing training at Gosford District Hospital in 1984. She has worked in hospitals, private nursing and palliative care, as well as a stint in Saudi Arabia. She qualified as a Naturopath at Nature Care College, Sydney and has completed a certificate in Female Sexual Health with NSW Family Planning. Ann-Mary has a particular interest in female sexual health from menarche to menopause. She ran a busy intravenous therapies clinic utilising chelation therapy and IV nutrient therapies, especially IV vitamin C. She has been a presenter and an education committee member and Education Co-ordinator for ACNEM (Australasian College of Nutritional & Environmental Medicine). Ann-Mary has also travelled extensively in Thailand, Malaysia and India supporting the development of integrative medical programs and colleges for doctors. She is now commencing study at Newcastle University planning to complete a Medical Degree.

Dr Peter Muzikants MB, BS (UNSW), FCPCA

Peter graduated in 1984 from the University of New South Wales with an MB and a BS, and has a Diploma of Laser Medicine and Dermatological from the Australasian College of Cosmetic Surgery. He has specialised in laser dermatology and aesthetic medicine since 1987. He has extensive experience with numerous dermatologic lasers for vascular, pigmentation and resurfacing. He is principal and director of Ada Aesthetic Medicine, a non-surgical, laser and aesthetic clinic with branches in Glebe, Sydney and Wollongong. He is on the advisory board of pharmaceutical companies for aesthetic use of neurotoxin and dermal fillers and is a national trainer for doctors in the use of dermal fillers and injectors and cosmetic neuromodulators. He has presented talks on lasers and non-surgical aesthetic procedures at many conferences and scientific meetings.

Suzie Hoitink

Suzie Hoitink is a health and skin expert, registered nurse, and founder of the Clear Complexions Clinics, which uses light based therapies. Suzie is a recipient of the 2012 ACT Telstra Business Women's Award and was a finalist in both the University of Canberra Distinguished Alumni Awards and the Nokia Innovation Award for developing the Clear Complexions Client Clinical Pathway. Suzie worked with a National Australia Working Party, instigated by the ACCS, to develop the first draft of the Professional Practice Standards and Scope of Practice for Aesthetic Nursing Practice in Australia. She is an in-demand authority on skin care, appearing on ABC and in national publications including Vogue, Harper's Bazaar, Cosmopolitan, Australian Women's Weekly, The Daily Telegraph and The Australian Nursing Journal. Suzie has also launched her own magazine, *Inner Confidence*.

Dr Kathy Gallagher

Dr Kathy Gallagher completed her medical degree at the University of Queensland in 1986. She worked as a general practitioner for over 25 years. She has had a special interest in cosmetic medicine, anti-ageing medicine and women's hormones for much of this time and has pursued further study in these fields. She regularly attends courses, events and conferences of interest. Opening Shine Cosmetic and Anti-Ageing Medicine Clinic in Clayfield, Brisbane in 2006 enabled her to combine these interests and pursue her passion for providing holistic solutions aimed at improving her patients' health and appearance.

Dr Bruce Williamson

Dr Williamson has worked in Skin Cancer and Cosmetic Medicine for over 20 years. He grew up on Sydney's northern beaches swimming, sailing and surfing, and had a lot of sun exposure in his early life. Consequently, he has developed a particular interest in combining the use of lasers with other technologies for rejuvenating sun-damaged skin. He established the Balgowlah Skin Cancer Clinic in 2000 and opened SkinSmart Medical Services in 2014 to offer a comprehensive range of non-surgical facial rejuvenation procedures.

Dr Jarrod Meerkin

Dr Jarrod Meerkin, an accredited Exercise Physiologist, began using DEXA in his Masters Research work and this progressed through to his PhD at QUT in Brisbane. Between 2002 and 2005 Dr Meerkin was a Senior Research Fellow at QUT in the School of Exercise and Sports Science, working with two of the leading researchers in the country in the obesity and exercise research domain. Through his extensive experience using DEXA in research Dr Meerkin saw a need in the consumer world for this important tool and established MeasureUp.

Elissa O'Keefe RN NP FFACNP MACN

Elissa O'Keefe is a Nurse Practitioner and the Director of Bravura Education: Exceptional laser e-learning for health professionals. She is passionate about delivering a superior learning experience and outcome to fit the needs and expectations of busy clinicians. She is a pioneer in the Australian healthcare landscape and the lead author of the Australasian College of Cosmetic Surgery's seminal document Professional Practice Standards and Scope of Practice for Aesthetic Nursing Practice in Australia (2015).

Tracey Beeby

Tracey Beeby has worked in the beauty industry for over 30 years. Her passion for the industry began when she was very young, and by the age of 18 she was managing a large salon and retail store. Tracey started her own business, The Skin Clinic, in North Ryde at just twenty-one, quickly gaining a reputation for raising the standards of excellence with endless hard work. She currently works as a global educator for Ultraceuticals.

Dr Glen Calderhead MSc PhD DrMedSci FRSM

Dr Glen Calderhead is an internationally recognised authority on the photobiological basics underpinning the application of lasers and light-emitting diodes in medicine and surgery, with four decades of experience in the field. With three books, several book chapters and over 100 publications in the peer-reviewed literature to his name, not to mention several hundred oral presentations, Dr Calderhead's name has become almost synonymous with light-emitting diode phototherapy, especially the term 'low level light therapy' and its acronym LLLT, for which he was responsible in 1988.

ADVISORY PANEL

Jenny Vallance, ACCS

Jenny has a strong background in the cosmetic medical field with more than 20 years' experience as a sales and marketing professional. She has been the managing director of both Collagen Corporation and Inamed, and uses her commercial skills in dealings with government, industry and Cosmetex, the latter now recognised internationally as the most prestigious cosmetic industry conference in Australia, attracting major overseas speakers and providing a program of excellence. Jenny is currently the general manager of the Australasian College of Cosmetic Surgery.

Matoyla Kollaras, Skin Factors

Matoyla started her career as an accountant for Pricewaterhouse, but life decided it had other ideas, and she moved into the skin care industry in 1994, founding Skin Factors Progressive Solutions. With a background in TCM, she is passionate about all things skin, integrative medicine, and epigenetics. Matoyla's health motto is 'We are the guardians of our genome.'

Shaun Connolly

Shaun has a background in sales and marketing in the hair, beauty, cosmeceutical and aesthetic equipment industries.

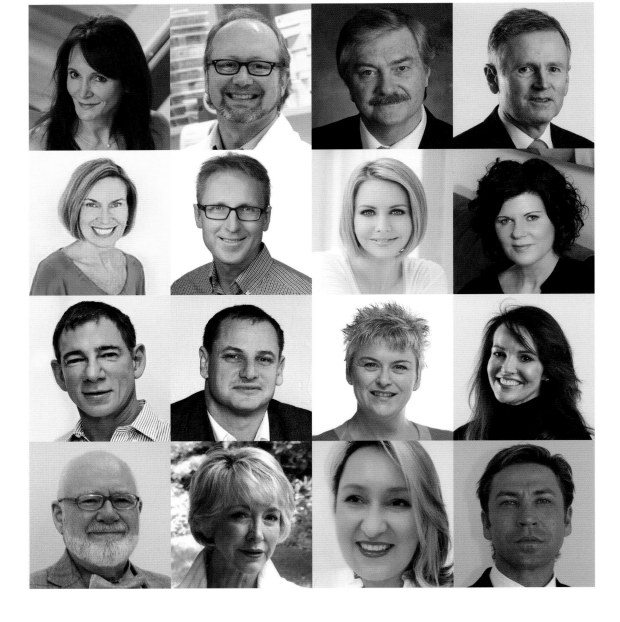

SLOW AGEING GUIDE TO SKIN REJUVENATION

L-R: Line 1 Kate Marie, Merlin Christopher Thomas, John Flynn, Geoffrey Heber
L-R: Line 2 Ann-Mary Hromek, Peter Muzikants, Suzie Hoitink, Kathy Gallagher
L-R: Line 3 Bruce Williamson, Jarrod Meerkin, Elissa O'Keefe, Tracey Beeby
L-R: Line 4 Glen Calderhead, Jenny Vallance, Matoyla Kollaras, Shaun Connolly

PREFACE

For many women, 'ageing well' means retaining their youthful skin. We use the appearance of our skin and, in particular, the skin on our face as a primary indicator of our health and vitality. To help achieve youthful skin, many women (and men) are turning to cosmetic medicine, using non-invasive or minimally invasive skin rejuvenation procedures.

It is not possible to turn back the clock or stop ageing, but this does not mean nothing can be done. Over the past twenty years we have learnt much about the science of skin and how to implement treatments that are evidence-based and can improve the health of our skin. While in the past many treatments were performed without any real understanding of the skin, today procedures are carefully designed to safely target specific elements of ageing skin to achieve certain results. From peptides and retinoids to lasers and radiofrequency, they all have specific roles and precise actions.

This book includes up-to-date information on the most recommended and effective cosmetic interventions that aim to improve the function of your skin. We believe that responsible choices start with gathering information from accurate and reviewed resources and from practitioners who are scientifically grounded in their work and the specifics of these procedures. This is what we aim to provide – accurate information so you can make the best decisions for your skin.

The biggest challenge facing cosmetic medicine is that technology often outstrips education and training, so be aware that while there are many clinics based around various new whizz-bang cosmetic technologies they may not know how to use them properly.

In many cases, it is the combined effects of multiple treatments that will make a real difference when it comes to combatting the effects of ageing on the skin. There are also limitations, side effects and costs. Sometimes selection of a treatment can be more complicated than it seems and so you need to make sure you go to practitioners who are medically trained, who keep up with the latest research, and who take a long-term view about skin care, in the same way your doctor takes a long term view of your overall health.

This book seeks to demystify skin rejuvenation procedures and technologies and put you safely on the path to ageing well. It covers the science of how ageing skin occurs and details the ways to slow its march.

Good things take time and effort, but getting the best information means making the best decisions to reach your goals.

Kate Marie & Professor Merlin Christopher Thomas

INTRODUCTION

Cosmetic medicine seems to polarise people and many women furtively go about addressing the health of their skin and appearance. They hide receipts for treatments from their husbands and deny they've had work done, even to close friends. The problem is that cosmetic medicine is often seen as an exercise in vanity and not a legitimate health practice, something that feeds off the youth-dominated culture we see all around us.

In fact, cosmetic medicine can be an important tool when it comes to preserving our health. We use it to look after our skin in the same way we care for our liver or other important body parts or organs. And not only does it have practical, beneficial results in and of itself, it can also inspire us in other areas of our life. Once we start looking great, we often want to stay that way and will seek to improve all aspects of our health care to retain that positive feeling. Our skin and its health is often a reflection of our internal health. By looking after our skin we also have a bridge into our total health. Rather than look at the skin in isolation, we need to address what we eat, how we think and address any internal health issues.

All too often the media perpetuates the idea that women have to look a certain way to be 'worthy' somehow, to have an appearance that fits a very limited set of criteria which are typically about appealing to men.

This is wrong, and not something we should be teaching girls and young women. We need to embrace womanhood in all stages of life, and seek to make ourselves feel and look good – for us.

It's all about intentions. If the use of cosmetic medicine feeds a part of us that we feel isn't 'good enough', then we start down a dangerous road. If, however, it makes you feel great and doesn't put you at risk then we can embrace its potential.

We have developed the SLOW philosophy to promote a positive approach to ageing. The AGELESS principles provide simple steps or considerations for when you are thinking about any skin treatment; whether that be diet, exercise, cosmetic procedures or skin care. Treatments and fads come and go and in the confusing and cluttered field of skincare products and treatments, there's much misinformation. It can be challenging to know how to make decisions and end up with products and treatments that actually work for you over the long term – and ensure you don't waste your hard-earned money.

When I (Kate) had my first mid-life crisis, I became fixated on how I looked, as I couldn't reconcile the difference between how I felt and who was looking back at me in the mirror. My familial frown line (affectionately known as 'the gutter' by my sister) had become a permanent fixture and I looked perpetually cross. I wasn't ready to sit and do nothing about it.

At the time, I was lucky enough to meet a doctor who helped me smooth things over (literally!) and I underwent Botox® treatment. It gave me a new lease on life; I had a renewed sense of confidence that those around me noticed straightaway.

Is it wrong, vain, or superficial to use a treatment such as anti-wrinkle injections? I don't think so. I don't see the need to let my outer organ, my skin, age any faster than it has to. This amazing organ has to last me for many years and I want to nurture, and protect it in the same way I'd do any asset. When I'm really old, I don't want to catch bits of loose skin on door handles and sharp edges, like many of the old women I cared for as a young nurse. I want my skin and its underlying structures to be adequately supported. I want to grow new collagen if I can. I want to encourage new layers of skin to grow and rid my system of redundant cells.

Many cosmetic skin treatments fit the slow ageing philosophy and are not simply quick fixes. They support sustainable, healthy ageing and help with the process of embracing ageing in a positive way.

Cosmetic medicine focuses not only on aesthetics, but aims to prevent ageing of our skin in a deeper way to promote better health. In the same way I look after my gut, brain and bones, I'm going to do whatever it takes to repair, remodel and improve my skin. If I look the better as a result, how lucky am I?

SECTION 1

CUTTING THROUGH THE CONFUSION

CHAPTER 1: THE SLOW AGEING APPROACH
CHAPTER 2: COSMETICS, COSMETIC MEDICINE AND COSMETIC (PLASTIC) SURGERY

We've developed the SLOW ageing philosophy and principles to help guide you toward the best possible decisions for you when it comes to your general and skin health. At the end of the book we also run through some simple steps on how to assess your options and how to select a practitioner that will help you achieve your skin rejuvenation goals.

Making an informed decision on cosmetic procedures can be challenging. Everyone has an opinion on what is the best approach, but this might not necessarily work for you. You need to be strategic and do your research. Fads and fashions come and go and most of us don't have the luxury of wasting money on something that doesn't work. You need to examine the evidence base to support specific treatments, make sure your practitioner is an expert and keeps up with the latest research and knowledge, and you also need to understand your own capacity to improve your skin – if you are a smoker, for example, then this will impact upon your choices and the results you can expect to achieve.

Cheap is not always the best, so be wary of going to practitioners that are trying to compete on price. Cosmetic medicine is not like buying a hair dye or getting your nails done. There might be serious consequences if you get into the hands of someone who doesn't know what they are doing. Laser work has long-term effects and in the wrong hands a laser can do some real damage. Look for practitioners that are motivated and invested in their professional education and who will keep you abreast of new ideas and technologies. They are the ones that will tell you to stop if necessary and not sell you unnecessary treatments.

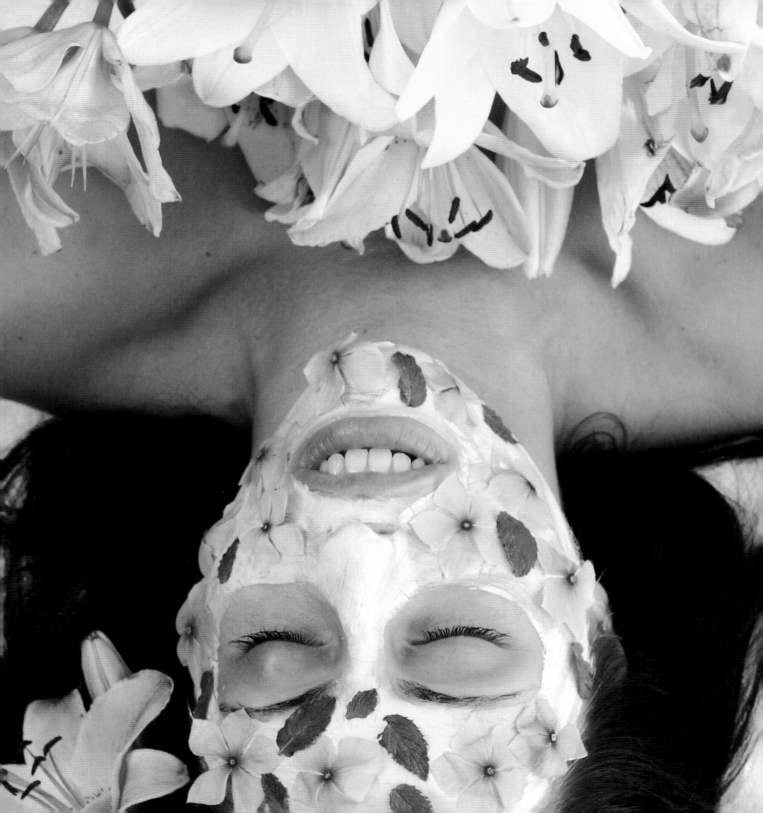

CHAPTER 01

THE SLOW AGEING APPROACH

Any health practice needs to be sustainable over the long term, and achieving optimal health for your skin is no different. The slow approach means being deliberate and strategic with all your health choices.

When we use the word 'SLOW', it doesn't mean procrastinating over your decisions or waiting until you have major problems before doing anything about them. 'SLOW' has a very specific meaning: taking your time to get the most value from any activity and decision.

Slow solutions set objectives that match your personal goals and capabilities. It is about taking stock of where you are now and being realistic about the health planning process and, in this case, planning for skin rejuvenation. This takes organisation as much as execution.

The best-known SLOW movement is the slow food movement. The slow food movement has used the acronym to mean:

S = Sustainable (not having an impact)

L = Local (not someone else's patch)

O = Organic (not mass produced)

W = Whole (not processed)

We've adapted the acronym to relate to maintaining optimal health as you age:

S = Strategic (becoming aware, investing time in planning and making the critical decisions required for you as an individual to slow the ageing process)

L = Long-term (to last for a lifetime)

O = Organised (implementing your plan against measurable objectives and investing effort into interventions that work for you)

W = Wilful (actions are undertaken and choices are made with full consciousness of their nature and effects)

SLOW is about taking time to find the connections in any experience and to savour their qualities. This is the same when it comes to selecting your food, being in a relationship or when it comes to dealing with the ageing process.

You don't want to be reckless and impulsive when your appearance, your health, and your happiness is at stake. Any cosmetic procedure, no matter how minimally invasive, always comes with some risk (what that is worthwhile in life doesn't?!) and this book aims to help you minimise it by empowering you to make informed decisions.

There are seven principles that characterise SLOW activities (we call them the AGELESS principles):

1. AWARENESS AND ENGAGEMENT

In this busy world, it's easy to fall asleep at the wheel and find yourself somewhere you didn't want to be. It's also easy to let someone else do the driving. SLOW puts you in control of your own choices. Much of your health depends on the choices you make (or fail to make). Making an informed decision requires time, research and careful deliberation. The best way to optimise the outcomes of a particular intervention is to be well informed. Learn as much as you can and constantly enrich your knowledge, which will give you the confidence to make the decision that's right for you.

2. GOAL SETTING BASED ON CLEAR AND REALISTIC EXPECTATIONS

Taking the long way to come to a decision does not mean an aimless meander. Slow solutions set objectives that match your personal goals and capabilities. They require planning, organisation and execution. SLOW is also about being realistic: being clear about what you are prepared to do, when, how, and most of all, why.

You want to understand what a specific cosmetic procedure can achieve and what it can't. The most common complaint about cosmetic medicine procedures is not bleeding or bruising, but unfulfilled expectations. Completely removing a wrinkle or achieving the 'perfect look' is not going to happen (very often). Cosmetic medicine is not a perfect science. It has real benefits but also limitations and you need to be aware of them. Cosmetic interventions can help delay or reduce the appearance of skin ageing, but it can never entirely stop the ageing process.

Discuss thoroughly with your practitioner and honestly inform him or her of issues that concern you the most. Ask questions and ask for clarification. The clearer, more realistic and flexible your expectations are, the more likely you are to be satisfied with the outcome of a treatment.

It also pays to consider your motivation for undertaking certain treatments, to reflect on how you feel about your appearance and what you really want to achieve. Unrealistic expectations of cosmetic procedures often extend beyond the surface of the skin. Cosmetic procedures can help you achieve a more positive self-image, but they will not save a marriage, or guarantee happiness. They will not secure a job promotion or a higher paying job. They will not remedy depression. This may sound silly, but it is not uncommon for some of us to have these goals tucked away at the back of our minds when approaching cosmetic treatments.

3. ELIMINATE THE NEGATIVE AND ACCENTUATE THE POSITIVE

The cosmetic industry positions 'getting old' as something to be avoided at all costs, or at the very least covered up. This is unrealistic and unnecessary. We want to slow ageing, not fear it. Attitude is the single most important factor in healthy ageing. It is possible to LOVE the ageing process. A positive attitude drives healthy behaviours and assures control over our own lives.

4. LONG-TERM AND SUSTAINABLE SOLUTIONS

Slow solutions are never a drastic change or a quick fix. They are not fads that claim 'success in only six weeks!'. Slow means something you can incorporate into your life on an ongoing basis. To commit to cosmetic medicine is to commit for the long term. There is no treatment that will provide all the answers in one visit. Almost always, multiple sessions, ongoing treatments and touch-ups are required for the best outcomes.

5. EXCLUSIVENESS SHOULD BE AVOIDED

Slow is not an alternative approach, but a complementary one. It acknowledges the roles different resources can play in reaching goals, as well as their limitations. There is no miracle 'cure-all' solution, but there are smaller answers that when put together add up to real results.

No matter what the advertising says, not every woman needs cosmetic medicine to maintain a youthful and healthy appearance. There are many things you can do to improve and maintain your appearance that don't include cosmetic procedures. Diet, exercise and good quality skincare all have real and long-lasting effects on the skin. For example, protecting your skin from excessive exposure to the sun can mean smoother, healthier skin in the long run. Cosmetic medicine can offer a range of highly effective interventions, but it works best in conjunction with a healthy lifestyle and an optimal skincare regime.

6. SUPPORT IS OUT THERE SO TAKE ADVANTAGE OF IT

Even if you're sitting in the driver's seat, it helps to have a guide. There are many cosmetic practitioners out there. The best of them are willing to act as 'coaches', rather than demand allegiance to particular strategies. Use their knowledge to help organise your thinking and explore the options available to achieve your objectives. Don't be afraid to look for support.

You need to know about the quality of the procedure you're getting and the expertise of the practitioner who's performing the procedure. After all, you are entrusting them your precious skin. Make sure to find a cosmetic practitioner who will respect your skin and take care of it as well as you do.

7. BE SELECTIVE

One size never fits all. A slow solution means choosing the right thing for you, in the right doses, at the right cost, at the right time and at the right pace.

Most women have cosmetic procedures to make them feel better about their appearance. If you choose to get a procedure, then do it for our own happiness, not for someone else's.

Planning to have a cosmetic procedure is not a decision that should be rushed. It is important to prepare well and put your plan into action at your own speed. Never commit to a cosmetic intervention if you have recently experienced a major life change or are experiencing emotional chaos. It's during these times that you can lose sight of your real objectives and there's a chance that you might consider a certain intervention for the wrong reason.

Are you emotionally ready? The physical changes occurring after some cosmetic procedures (positives and negatives) can have a real effect on your emotions. No matter how small, changes on the outside can have a tremendous effect on how you feel on the inside. Self-image is one of the biggest regulators of our emotions, so take your time to find out if you are really ready.

The decision to opt for any cosmetic intervention is a personal one. There are many resources available to help make your decision including books (like this one), friends who have had procedures and cosmetic specialists. However, nobody will understand the importance of your goals and your capacity to achieve them better than you do.

Don't let anyone talk you into doing anything you are uncomfortable with. Keep in mind that your practitioner is tasked to guide you and to provide unbiased information about what might be the most appropriate interventions for you, and let you know of any potential risks and side effects. They should not make decisions for you, as you should always have the final say when it comes to your skin. It is also important to know your own limits. Whether these limits are financial, emotional, or related to pain tolerance, respect them. Don't be blinded to who you really are by some slick salesman.

The point of cosmetic medicine is to show who you are, not to turn you into someone else.

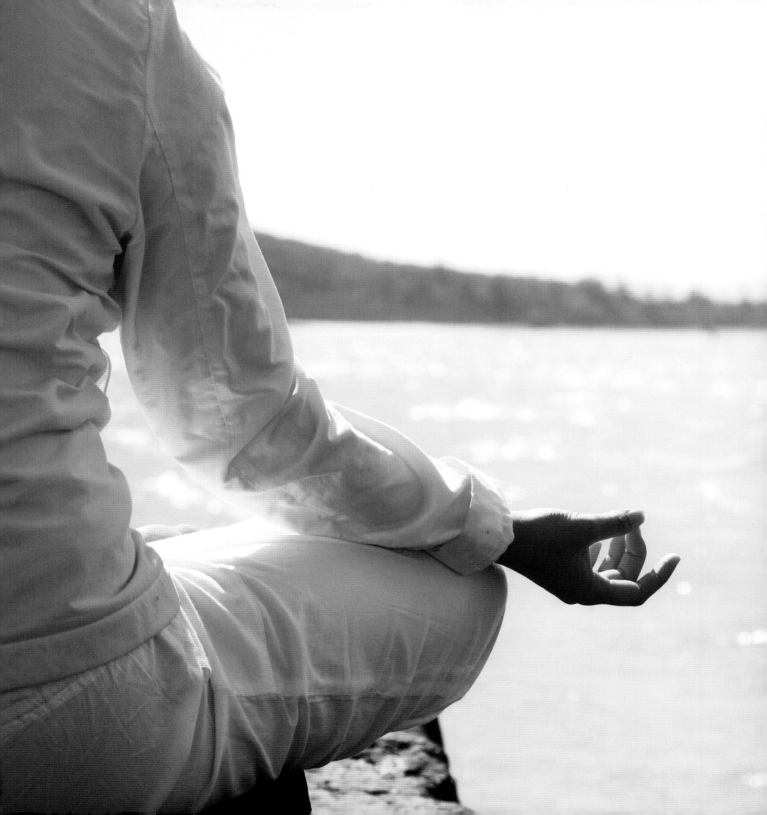

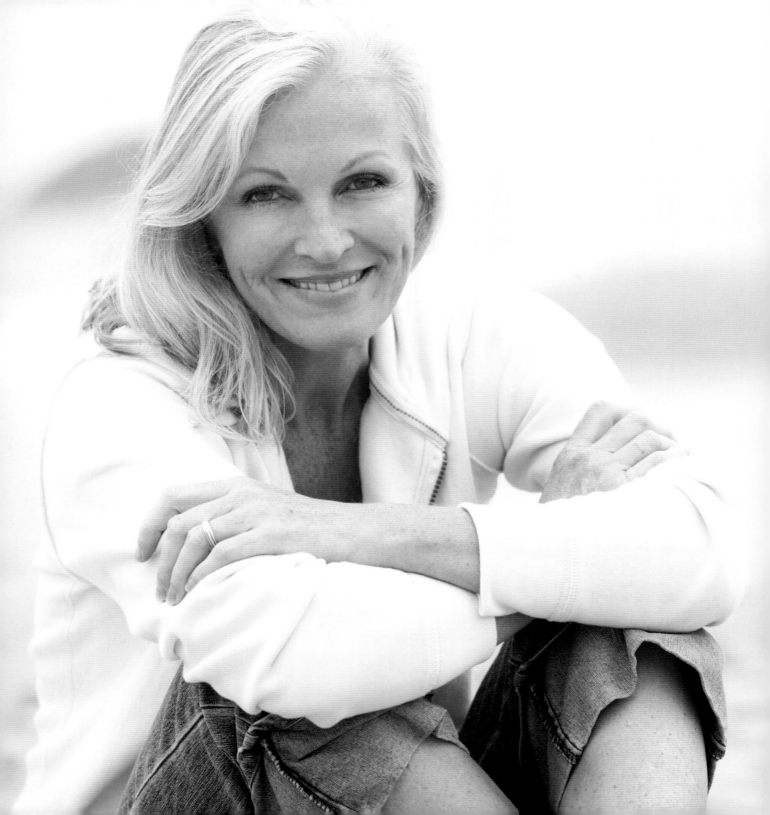

CHAPTER 02
COSMETICS, COSMETIC MEDICINE AND COSMETIC (PLASTIC) SURGERY

Cosmetics is an enormous industry whose aim is to reduce or mask the appearance of ageing. There are millions of products that are applied everyday by billions of women around the world for cleansing, beautifying or otherwise altering the appearance of the skin. These are known as cosmetics or makeup and include everything from highlights to lipstick. Their wares usually fill the ground floor of large department stores and chemist shops. A cosmetician (also known as a cosmetologist or makeup artist) is a professional who provides these cosmetic treatments for clients. Cosmetics are not medicines. Their effect does not continue any longer than we wear the product and does not lead to long lasting alterations in our appearance. Their effects are often said to be 'only skin deep', as they sit on the skin's surface.

COSMETIC MEDICINE WHEN CORRECTLY EXECUTED HAS INTEGRITY

Cosmetic medicine, in contrast, is a medical discipline and should only be undertaken by registered practitioners. Cosmetic medicine includes a range of procedures for which robust evidence exists regarding their safety and effectiveness. The most common procedures include resurfacing, photo-rejuvenation, and a range of injectables (all of which will be discussed in this book). The common goal of every cosmetic medicine intervention is to physically change the skin to create a more vibrant and youthful look.

A number of topical agents are also available that act to change the appearance of the skin, rather than simply camouflaging it. These are known as cosmeceuticals and are discussed in Section 6. In this category are a diverse range of products including moisturisers, exfoliants, antioxidants, retinoids, hormones and peptides. Many of these agents are available over the counter and are widely used in conjunction with cosmetic products to broaden their utility. However, some cosmeceuticals require a prescription, especially in the high doses required to have the optimal effects.

BENEFITS OF COSMETIC MEDICINE

Most cosmetic medicine is minimally invasive and can be performed either without sedation or with a local anaesthetic. Cosmetic surgery, in contrast, is highly specialised, requires dedicated practitioners and specialist clinics, and are mostly performed under general anaesthesia. The best known cosmetic surgery procedures include nose reshaping, liposuction, breast augmentation, nasal and eyelid surgery, and facelifts.

Surgical intervention is widely believed to be the gold standard for combatting the changes ageing has on the face and the body. While it can achieve dramatic improvements in the appearance of our skin, but it has a number of disadvantages. Many women feel that the prolonged recovery time, the significant expense, and the risk of side effects represent major barriers. It is thus often felt to be a choice of last resort. Most women would prefer less invasive, less expensive options with lower risk and shorter (or no) recovery times.

There are now many products and procedures that are touted as 'non-surgical options to cosmetic surgery', including alternatives to liposuction, facelifts and augmentation surgery. This does not they can do the same job. The big changes that can be achieved by surgery can rarely be matched by other cosmetic procedures. In the right patients, with mild to moderate skin problems, the subtler effects of cosmetic medicine can come to the fore. Rather than waiting to be 'bad enough to need a facelift', many women feel far more comfortable intervening earlier when the treatment is simple and non-invasive to create a long-term program of rejuvenation and skin maintenance.

The increasing use and expertise with non-surgical cosmetic procedures has remarkably broadened the use of such therapies, from focal touch-ups to more comprehensive protocols that combine different treatments. Even within the last five years, standardisation of treatment protocols and their delivery have significantly improved not only how well the treatments work, but also how predictably they work. In addition, greater understanding of how interventions actually work has led to the development of much more selective interventions that produce less collateral injury to the skin, while still ensuring the desired results. The development of fractional lasers for laser resurfacing is an example of one such advance (see Section 8).

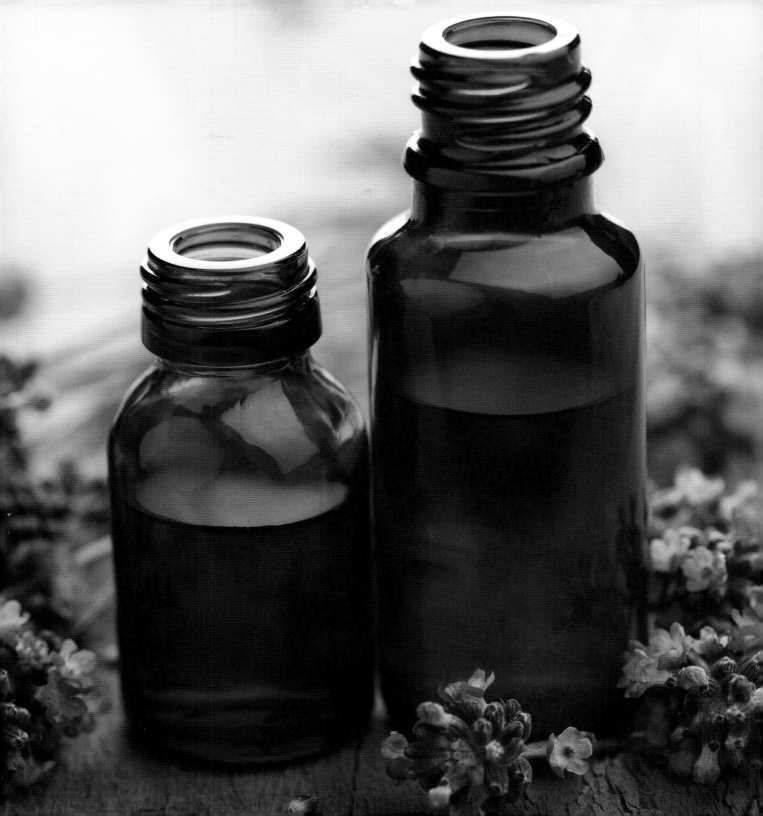

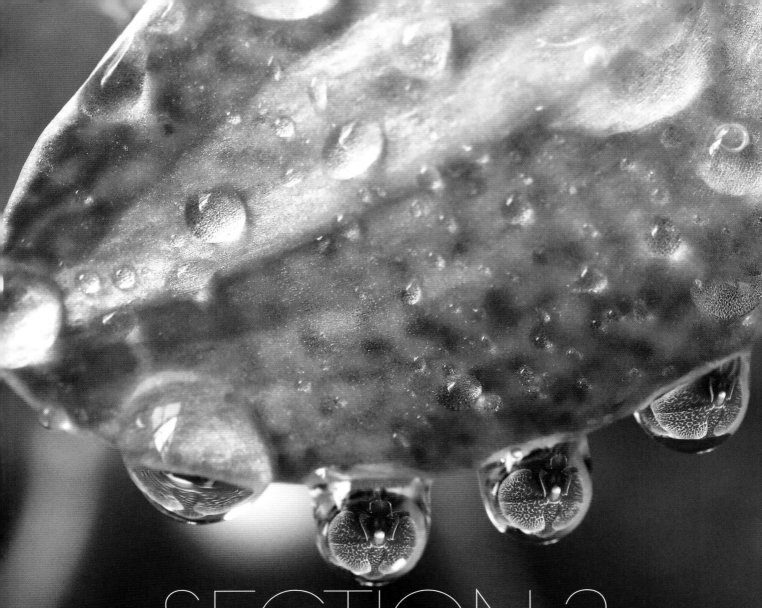

SECTION 2:
WHAT HAPPENS TO THE SKIN AS IT AGES?

CHAPTER 3: THE EPIDERMIS
CHAPTER 4: THE DERMIS (INNER SKIN)
CHAPTER 5: THE SUBDERMIS

To better understand what can realistically be done about wrinkles, lines, spots and other aspects of the ageing process, it is important to know how the skin works and how it changes as we age.

At its most basic, skin is your outer covering and the first point of contact your body has with the outside environment. It has to defend our insides against sunlight, pollution, bacteria, smoke, climate, drying out, getting wet, etc. For this it suffers greatly.

Human skin is composed of multiple layers, each of which serves a particular function that affects its appearance. Put simply, your skin can be viewed as three layers: the epidermis (the outermost layer of the skin), the dermis (the inner layer beneath the epidermis) and the subdermis (the fatty layer underneath which is not exactly part of the skin but is an important factor in how our skin looks).

There are a number of different components within each of these layers. There are also interactions between the layers, but this simple division into three is useful, as cosmetic treatments will generally aim to target one of them. For example, peels and microdermabrasion will focus on the outer epidermis. Non-ablative lasers and radiofrequency will target the deeper dermis, while lipolysis will get under the skin to the subdermis. Knowing these three layers and what they do makes it easier to understand what cosmetic treatments can do for you and what might be the best option(s) for your personal needs.

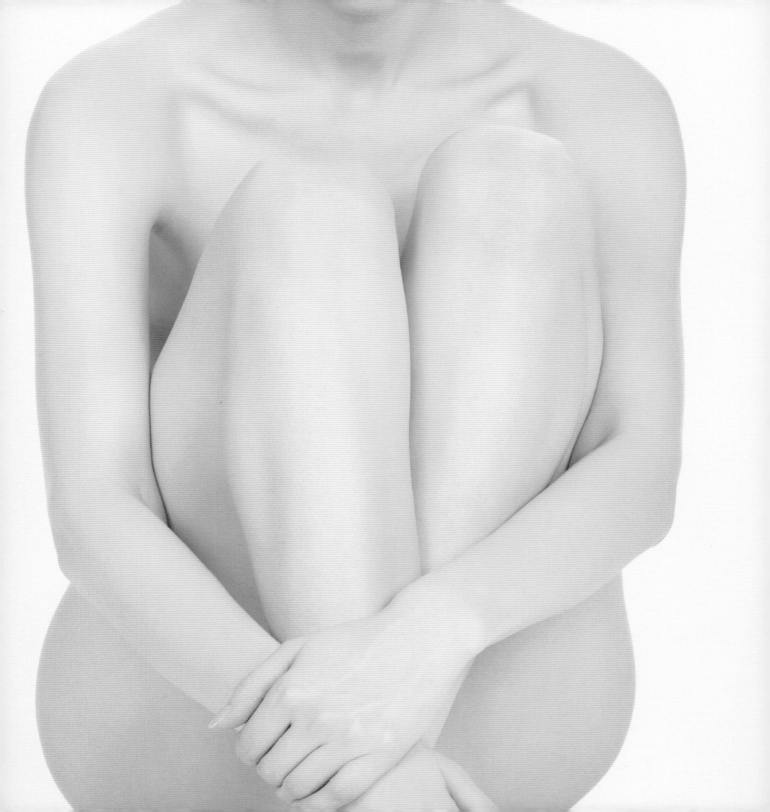

CHAPTER 03

THE EPIDERMIS

The epidermis is the outermost layer of the skin. It is thin, like the peel of an apple, but it is anything but superficial. The epidermis performs two major functions. First and foremost, the epidermis is a barrier to stop bad things (such as bugs, toxins and radiation) from getting inside the body. It also stops all the important parts inside from drying out.

The epidermis is essentially a stack of skin cells known as keratinocytes. From top to bottom, the epidermis is about fifty cells deep, spanning about a tenth of a millimetre.

WE NEED TO ENCOURAGE CELL TURNOVER

Each day, about one new layer of skin cells is made on the inside of the epidermis and each day one layer on the outside is shed. This process is often described as a conveyer belt, but is more akin to one of those executive toys where one silver ball strikes at one end and displaces the ball at the other end. Either way, every six to seven weeks you have an entirely new epidermis.

New skin cells are big, full of moisture and actually shaped a bit like bricks. As the cells are forced toward the surface of the skin by the constant generation of new cells in the deepest layers underneath them, they get farther from the nutrients they need to survive. They become progressively thinner and flatter until eventually they die and become keratin, a hard protein that provides some of the skin's resilience. The outermost part of the epidermis (known as the stratum corneum) consists of almost thirty layers of interconnected dead cells. However, these layers are not immune to the constant evolution of the skin and they are shed as more and more new cells push up from below.

As we get older, the turnover and replacement of the epidermis slows as nutrient delivery to the skin declines. As such, grazes and cuts (as well as any cosmetic treatments) take a lot longer than when we were young. At the same time, slower skin turnover means a slower rate of shedding the old skin, causing a pile-up of dead skin on the surface. This makes the surface look and feel dry, rough, flaky and generally dull in appearance. The pattern of growth is also less streamlined as we get older. This means that some areas grow at faster rates than others, making older skin look somewhat scaly as cells clump together in some areas but not in others. This may also contribute to the appearance of fine lines.

If your skin looks and feels old because the turnover of skin cells in the epidermis is slow, then the solution is obvious. Stimulate skin turnover to look younger! This is precisely what many cosmetic treatments do. For example, if you have a light (superficial) peel, laser or dermabrasion treatment, it removes some or all of the outer layer of dead cells from the epidermis. This procedure is also called 'resurfacing', because this is exactly what it does (see section 9).

SKIN MOISTURISING FACTORS

As noted above, the outer layer of the skin is mostly dead cells. The longer skin cells have been dead, the drier they look and feel. This is one reason why, as we get older, the slower turnover of skin cells leads to a dry-feeling skin, but it is not the only reason. The other thing that makes up the outer layer of the skin and gives it its moisture-retaining qualities is the presence of natural moisturising factors, such as lipids and glycosaminoglycan (also known as GAGs). Over time as we age, these elements can also diminish.

> **Lipids.** Lipids make up about twenty percent of the outer layer of the epidermis. If you think of the cells of the epidermis as the bricks, then lipids are the mortar surrounding them. The lipids hold the cells in place and stop water or other potentially damaging elements from sneaking through. The most important of the lipids are called ceramides, which link with other components to form a virtually impenetrable barrier to water. Unfortunately, ceramides can decline by as much as two-thirds in ageing skin, compromising the protective function of the skin as well as lowering its moisture content. Many anti-ageing creams include emollients, which partly act to replace missing lipids and restore the barrier to contaminants. Some creams even contain ceramides or lactic acid, which can help stimulate lipid generation.

> **Glycosaminoglycans (GAGs).** The moisture-retaining properties of the skin are largely determined by its amount of GAGs. Like a sponge, GAGs can hold up to a thousand times their dry weight in water. When our skin gets older, the content of GAGs in the epidermis declines, therefore so does the skin's ability to retain water. This makes our skin both look and feel thinner, as well as become more prone to drying out. This is one reason that being in dry environments (e.g. on a plane) has a significant effect on the appearance of ageing skin.

Many skin creams and cosmetics contain GAGs. Unfortunately, our GAGs cannot be replaced by creams or lotions. AHAs (alpha-hydroxy acids) and tretinoin are well known to increase epidermal and dermal hyaluronic acid concentration, another element that promotes skin hydration. Retinol does this as well. Other moisturisers can be used to restore and enhance the moisture-retaining properties of the epidermis. These are called humectants and are discussed in Chapter 18.

THE MANTLE

On the very outer surface of our skin is a thin film called sebum. It is composed of oil, wax, acids and a complex mixture of many other chemicals, including antioxidants, natural antibiotics and pheromones. It is not sweat, which is mostly salt water rather than oil. This film of oil is often called the mantle, because like a shawl, it is there for protection.

Sebum is secreted by sebaceous glands through tiny pores in the skin. The cells of these glands make sebum by bursting open and dying, so what coats our skin is actually the disintegrated remnants of dead cells. Luckily, there is normally a healthy regeneration as new cells are constantly being made, replacing the old ones.

A number of different factors affect how much oil we have sitting on the surface of our skin, including our gender, hormones, diet, ethnicity and climate. Some people have naturally oily skin, especially across the forehead, nose and chin (known as the 'T zone'). This can make their skin look shiny, and feel unclean. Too much oil can also block pores, which leads to acne and blackheads.

Another important factor that affects the oiliness of our skin is age. In fact, levels of oil on our skin slowly decline as we get older. This is because as we get older cell turnover slows and the rate of cell bursting and oil production also slows to stay in balance. A lack of skin surface oils can make older skin more vulnerable to the drying effects of detergents and soaps.

To compensate for reduced sebum production, the size of our pores also increases as we get older. Bigger pore openings can sometimes give an unpleasant 'orange peel' look to the skin. Many anti-ageing cosmetics contain astringents, like witch hazel, that temporarily cause pores to shrink, making the skin look and feel smoother.

WHAT CAUSES AGE SPOTS?

Living in the deep layers of the epidermis are pigment cells known as melanocytes. These cells make the dark pigment called melanin, which they then transfer to other skin cells, to provide them with resistance against the harmful effects of sunlight. Melanin gives our skin its natural colour. People with fair skin make and have melanin in their skin, but people with naturally dark skin have much more of it.

As we get older, it's quite common for our skin to develop blotchy, uneven areas that appear darker than the surrounding skin. These are commonly known as age spots, or sun spots as they are often most obvious on areas of our skin that have been consistently or excessively exposed to sunlight, such as the face, shoulders, hands and arms. Age spots look a bit like freckles and both can be triggered by sunlight. However, freckles will increase in number and become darker with more sun exposure, as pigment cells (melanocytes) make more pigment in response to excess sunlight. By contrast, within age spots there are simply more pigment cells making a normal amount of pigment, so once they form, they can hang around regardless of how much sun we subsequently get. Age spots can also appear in areas not exposed to much sun. Age spots can affect any skin type, but are a particular problem for paler Asian women.

Age spots are thought to appear because, although the number of pigment cells in our skin slowly declines as we get older (by between 10 and 20 percent each decade), this can be a patchy process, leaving islands of pigment cells desperately trying to make up for losses elsewhere. This leads to some areas looking darker than the surrounding skin and so giving the skin a blotchy appearance.

Because the problem of age spots is a result of more melanin producing cells in a particular area, cosmetic treatments tend to try and even out the skin's melanin content to make it appear less blotchy. This is usually achieved with pigment lasers or light therapy that specifically target melanin.

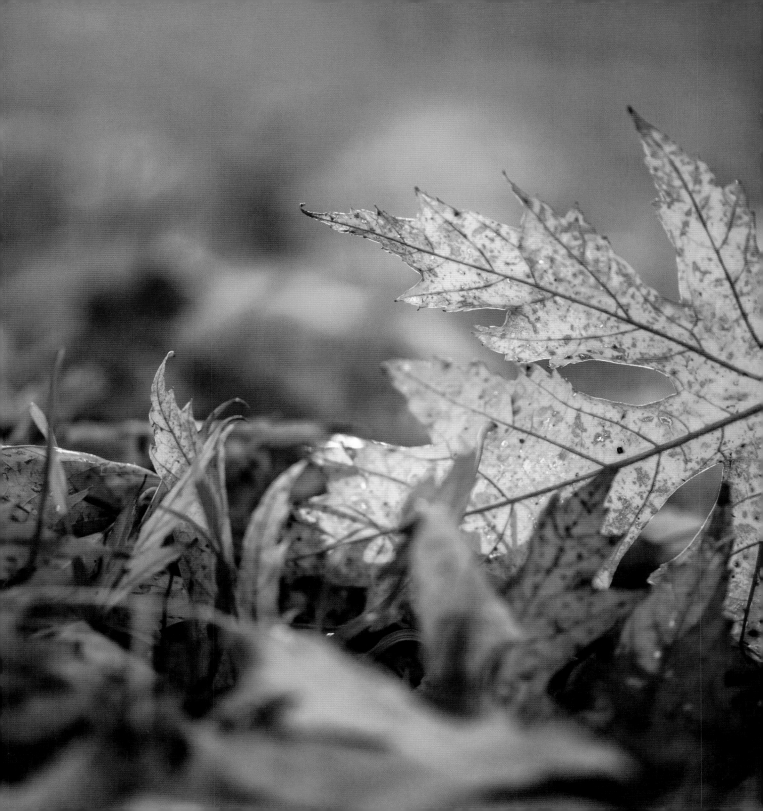

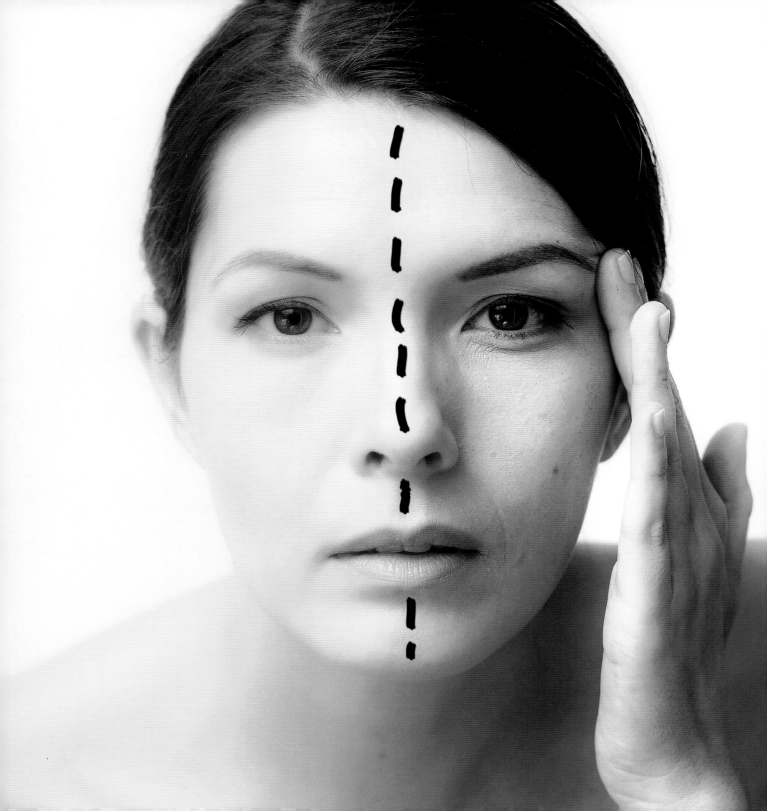

CHAPTER 04

THE DERMIS (INNER SKIN)

The most significant ageing processes, in terms of skin appearance, occur below the epidermis in the layer of the skin called the dermis. This layer is what determines whether our skin feels thick or thin to us. On average the dermis is two to three millimetres thick, but some areas are naturally thinner than others. For example, the skin located around our eyes and on our eyelids is only around half a millimetre thick.

Our dermis gets thicker during childhood and adolescence, reaching its peak in our twenties, but after that it steadily becomes thinner. On average, it is thinner by about a third by the time we reach eighty years of age.

THE MATRIX

The dermis is filled with skin cells whose chief job is to make lots of connective tissue (also known as matrix). This matrix is essentially the organised scaffold that holds the skin together. The most important matrix proteins are collagen, elastin and proteoglycans. These are highly specialised components that provide mechanical support for the skin and much of the strength, resilience and elasticity of skin.

The production of matrix in our skin slowly declines as we get older. For example, the collagen content of our skin declines by about one percent per year of our adult life. This is partly because there are fewer cells, turning over more slowly and so making less matrix.

Not only is there less matrix as we get older, old matrix will not pull itself together as well, compounding the problem. Instead of being a delicate organised scaffold that provides support to the skin and a nice place for our skin cells to live, the main structural proteins of the matrix slowly deteriorate under the ravages of sunlight, smoking, oxidative stress and the other elements.

Our skin is programmed to heal. Damaged skin makes more enzymes (called matrix metalloproteinases or MMPs) to clean up the mess, by breaking down and turning over dysfunctional matrix proteins. But healing is never perfect, and is increasingly less perfect as we get older, so every little bit of damage leaves behind a few more fragmented and disorganised fibres.

As we age the dermis has less ability to stretch and becomes less elastic. When pressed, it no longer springs back into position; instead older skin sags and forms furrows. For example, as the underlying support for the skin over our brow declines, it can slowly but progressively droop (known as ptosis), leaving a sagging uneven brow. The bags under our eyes can get bigger and deeper, and even our nose gets a little longer. This is chiefly because the dermis and the matrix it manufacturers is not doing its job as well as it did when we were younger.

WRINKLES AND CRINKLES

We all get wrinkles as we get older. Wrinkles happen in very specific places because of the way our skin is stretched by movement. They are usually most obvious on our face because the facial muscles are among the most active in the whole of our body, constantly stretching and contracting our skin. The most common types of wrinkles include:

> **Worry lines** (also known as forehead creases). Horizontal lines on our forehead that makes us look like we are stressed all the time.
> **Frown lines** (also known as glabellar or furrow lines). Vertical lines between our eyebrows that look like the number eleven.
> **Crow's feet.** Splaying creases around the outer corners of the eyes that make us look like we are squinting.
> **Bunny lines** (also known as nasal wrinkles). These are wrinkles that form over the bridge of the nose and between our eyes, and can give the appearance that we are twitching our nose or squinting.
> **Nasolabial folds.** Lines that run from the sides of the nose down to the corners of the mouth and separate the cheek from the upper lip. We all have lines here, but they get deeper and more prominent as we get older. These are one of the earliest signs of ageing, which usually begin to reveal themselves between the late thirties and mid-forties.
> **Lipstick lines** (also known as labial lines or smoker's lines). Lines over our top lip that make us look like we are pursing our lips.
> **Oral commissures** (also known as mouth lines). Like crow's feet only around the corners of the mouth rather than the eyes.
> **Marionette lines.** These are lines than run downwards from the corners of our mouth, and can make us look a little like a puppet when we speak.
> **Parenthesis lines** (also known as smile lines).
> **Chin dimples and creases** (also known as mental creases).

Some wrinkles can really only be seen when our face is moving, as when squinting or smiling. These are often called 'expression lines' or 'dynamic wrinkles'. These wrinkles can make a face more expressive as we get older, and are often deliberately accentuated by stage actors. Sometimes this is not a good thing – especially when we aren't really that stressed, angry or worried. Getting rid of wrinkles is the most common cosmetic procedure and is used to target either:

> **Static wrinkles.** Wrinkles that are somewhat fixed on the face and don't change much with facial expression.
> **Crinkles or fine lines.** These often appear as crosshatched lines, like on aluminium foil, which starts out smooth and flat on the roll, but any use and it gets all crinkly.

As most wrinkles and lines are caused by reduced elasticity in the dermis, the logical treatment is to use cosmetic procedures that improve its elasticity. Typically, such treatments work by breaking down the disorganised matrix and stimulating the production of healthy, organised collagen. Because it's the dermis we are talking about, with the exception of retinoids and AHAs little if anything gets past the outer epidermis. Therefore, few skin creams will get to where they are really needed, let alone help it to make more collagen, and as a result most wrinkle creams don't work.

By contrast, newer cosmetic treatments including laser, radiofrequency and pulse light therapy are able to specifically target the dermis. Fillers and volumisers are also popular wrinkle treatments, and act to increase the thickness and resilience of the dermis in particular sites (like underneath wrinkles). All of these treatments work best when combined with injections that relax the muscles that express lines and wrinkles on the face (see chapter 22). This gives the skin a chance to remodel without simply wrinkling up again under the force of facial expression.

VISIBLE BLOOD VESSELS

The dermis also has a rich supply of blood vessels, which provide the nutrients for all layers of the skin as well as contributing to its colour. With age, the number of these small vessels progressively declines, contributing to the slower turnover of skin cells. At the same time, it means that older skin feels cooler to the touch and is less able to cope with changes in temperature. With less support from the dermis, the blood vessels themselves also become more fragile, which can lead to easier bruising.

TELANGIECTASIA

As the matrix becomes weaker with age, blood vessels situated throughout the dermis are also more prone to becoming stretched. Sometimes skin blood vessels, instead of going away, become more visible as we get older. These are known as telangiectasia and may appear as tiny red, purple or blue spots. Telangiectasia are common on the face, particularly on the nose and cheeks, especially in women with fair skin. It is easy to tell they are a blood vessel because when you press them hard enough to stop the blood flow, they will temporarily disappear, and then slowly refill and reappear after you let go. Fortunately, small telangiectasia can be easily treated using lasers that specifically target visible blood vessels with little or no damage to surrounding skin tissues.

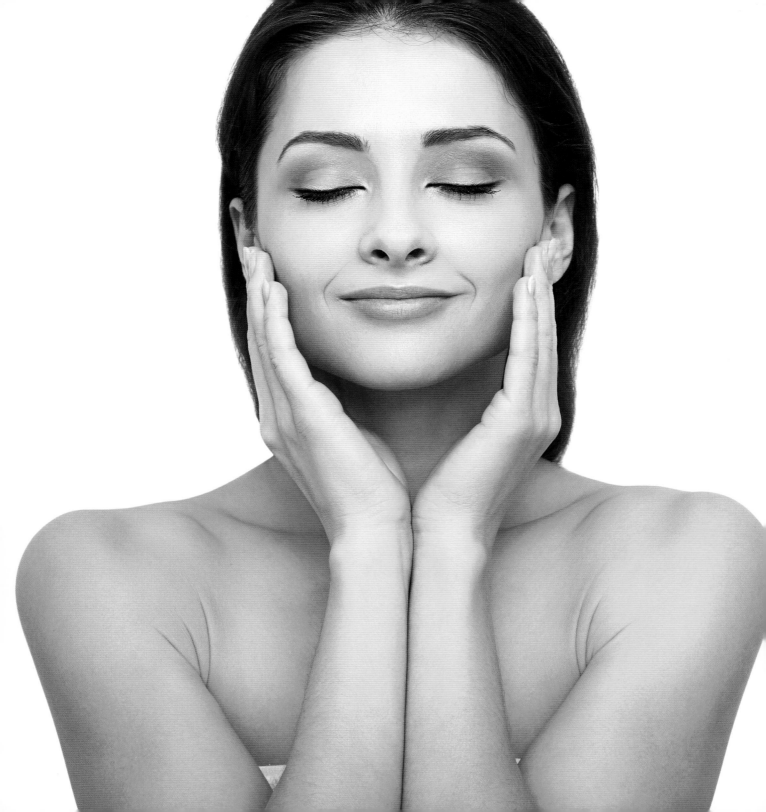

CHAPTER 05

THE SUBDERMIS

Changes in the tissues underneath the skin also significantly impact upon our appearance. This layer of tissue is called the subdermis or subcutaneous layer. It consists mainly of fat cells known as adipocytes. These fat cells function as cushioning shock absorbers for the skin as well as insulators against heat loss.

LOSS OF FAT LEADS TO FACIAL CHANGES

With age, our skin loses its fatty cushions in some places but not in others. Although our waists and thighs are often expanding, fat deposits under the skin in the cheeks, in the shins and the back of the hands tend to reduce in volume.

In particular, redistribution of fat in the face changes the shape of our faces as we age, making it appear more hollow, especially under the eyes and cheeks, and over the forehead, temples and chin. At the same time, fat increasingly accumulates under the skin near the brow, jaws, chin, and neck. This can make an older face appear more 'squared off' or 'unbalanced' compared to the defining arcs and lines and the generally more angular shape of a younger face.

Recognising that it is loss of fat volume under our skin that is changing the way we look gives us an obvious solution: put some volume back. This is called augmentation, and is why many cosmetic regimes include fillers and volumisers. Some treatments also aim to directly put fat back where it should be, or blast it out of where it shouldn't. This is called sculpturing, and is emerging as a popular cosmetic treatment.

DARK CIRCLES UNDER THE EYES

Dark circles under our eyes are also more common as we age. They can make us look as though we are sad, tired or stressed. Most people blame a lack of sleep or frequent rubbing of tired eyes as the probable reason. Certainly, dark circles (and puffy eyes) are worse first thing in the morning. This has led some people to suggest that the dark colour is caused by blood pooling in the veins just under the skin when lying flat in bed.

Most dark circles don't actually result from the skin becoming dark. What starts out as pretty flat when we are young, becomes progressively hollowed with age, as the fat in the subdermis rearranges itself. This causes the tear trough to increasingly be prone to become lost in shadows, hence the dark circles. At the same time, the dermis and subdermis directly under our eyes becomes thinner, revealing some of the darker blood rich muscles below the eyes. Dark circles can also result from conditions such as dermal melanin deposition, post inflammatory hyperpigmentation secondary to atopic or allergic contact dermatitis, periorbital oedema, superficial location of vasculature, and shadowing due to skin laxity

Many of the best-known cures for dark circles under the eyes actually work by temporarily tightening the skin and/or driving the blood away from the skin's surface. Among the most famous remedies include wet, cold tea bags, rose water and – everyone's favourite – cucumber slices. Sadly, none of these are a long-term solution. Tightening technologies like laser, radiofrequency and fillers have all been used with some success in people troubled by dark circles under their eyes.

INCREASED CELLULITE HAPPENS WITH AGE

Cellulite is the unsightly dimpling and lumpiness of the skin, mostly over our thighs, buttocks and hips. It occurs in almost all women to a greater or lesser extent at some point. It is more common as we get older, and particularly as we get fatter.

Cellulite is thought to be caused by changes in the boundary between the dermis and the fat underlying it in the subdermis. Normally, there is a pretty clear demarcation, but the appearance of cellulite means that some fat has squeezed up and into the connective tissue layers of the dermis. This is likely due to changes in the skin's blood flow, inflammation and scarring.

To reduce the amount and severity of cellulite, the most obvious solution is to reduce the amount of fat under our skin. This can be achieved surgically with liposuction, which literally sucks the fat away from under the skin. However, newer, non-invasive treatments that target the fat under the skin also work, including fat-busting lasers, ultrasound, cryosculpting and other technologies. The use of these treatments is commonly known as 'contouring' (see chapter 12).

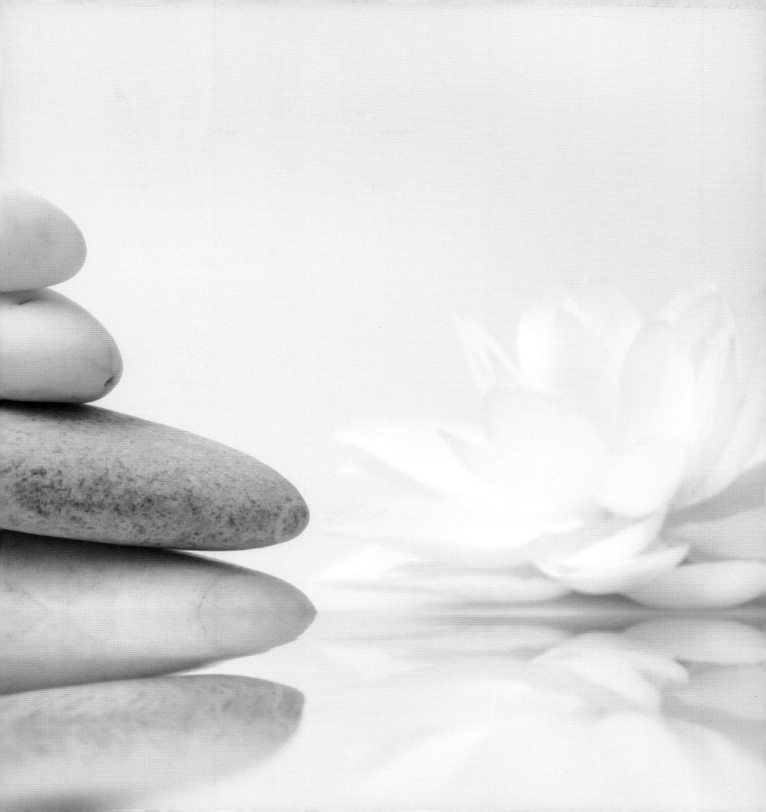

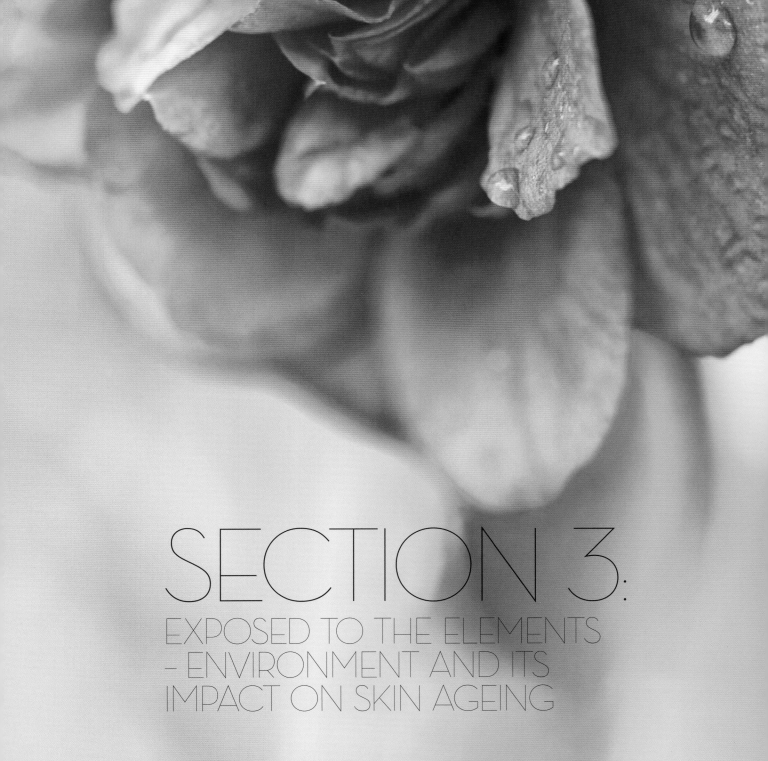

SECTION 3:
EXPOSED TO THE ELEMENTS – ENVIRONMENT AND ITS IMPACT ON SKIN AGEING

CHAPTER 6: THE SUN – ENEMY OF THE SKIN
CHAPTER 7: SMOKE AND AIR POLLUTION
CHAPTER 8: OTHER ENVIRONMENTAL IMPACTS ON AGEING SKIN

The ageing process is most easily appreciated in the weather beaten faces of people who spend most of their lives outdoors, like farmers, mountaineers, Eskimos or desert dwellers. Their wrinkles tend to be deeper and their skin thick and unevenly pigmented. In essence, they typically look older than their years. Their weathered skin is an extreme example of long-term exposure to an extreme climate.

However, we are all exposed to the weather to some extent, and without protection this will eventually age our skin.

The importance of this weathering can be understood by examining our wrinkles. They happen to all of us, but not at the same time, in the same way or to the same extent. We may be as old as our friends from school, but we don't necessarily look the same age.

As discussed in the previous section, ageing slowly undermines our skin, meaning it becomes less elastic and less resilient, leading to creases, lines and wrinkles. Time is not the only element involved; sunlight, smoking, pollution, hormones, stress and many other factors can also injure our skin. With each natural shock, our skin carries a tiny legacy, which helps transform it ever so slowly from young to old.

However, by limiting exposure or reducing modifiable factors concerned with environment, we can allow ageing to slowly take its time. Ageing is not something we want to help along or speed up!

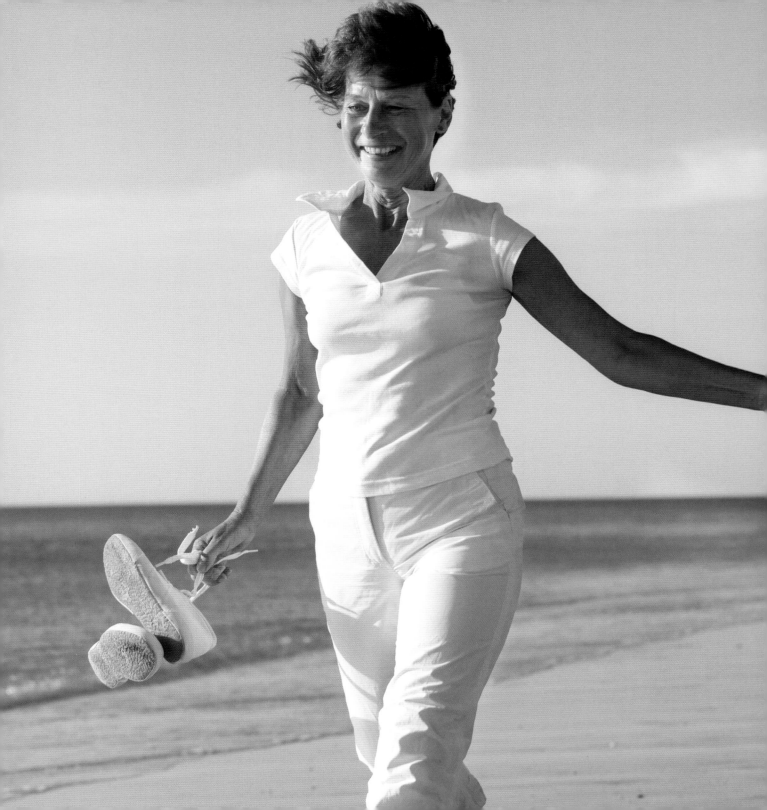

CHAPTER 06
THE SUN – ENEMY OF THE SKIN

Getting out in the sun is an essential component of maintaining good health, but it can come at a cost to our skin. If continuous exposure of our skin to the natural elements causes wrinkles and spots, then the most important of these elements has to be sunlight.

Four out of every five wrinkles and most of the unwanted spots on our face are due to sun exposure. In fact, sunlight is responsible for most of the visible changes in our skin's appearance as we get older. When we despair about our wrinkles and lines, roughness, mottled pigmentation and spots, we need not look further than our time under the sun for their probable cause.

The cumulative effects of sunlight on our skin can be seen if we look at the sun-exposed skin on our neckline and compare it to the less-exposed skin next to it on our chest. The exposed skin looks different. It tends to have more wrinkles, mottled colour, prominent small blood vessels and a leathery feel. This is quite different from the skin next to it that has been protected from the sun, which although it is exactly the same age, is characteristically much smoother and unblemished.

SUNLIGHT'S EFFECT ON THE SKIN

Every time we go out in daylight, our skin is irradiated with light coming from the sun. Sunlight is just light energy travelling over a spectrum of different wavelengths. On average, about half is invisible infrared radiation, while about a third is light that we can see. The remaining solar energy is short-wavelength ultraviolet radiation. Ultraviolet light reaching our skin is further divided into UVA and UVB (sometimes called long-wave and short-wave UV, respectively).

UVB is more damaging to our skin than UVA. In high doses UVB will literally kill the epidermal layer of our skin, resulting in sunburn. However, UVA penetrates much deeper than UVB into the dermis layer of the skin. In addition, our skin gets at least twenty times more exposure to UVA than UVB, so what it lacks in strength it more than makes up in quantity.

This is because the protective ozone layer in the earth's atmosphere blocks out over ninety percent of UVB, but allows most of the UVA to get through. (There is also a UVC light, but this doesn't penetrate the earth's atmosphere at all.)

Because of the key role of the atmosphere in determining UVB penetration, our exposure to UVB is quite variable and dependent on a host of atmospheric factors. For example, UVB radiation is greatest in summer. Most of the day's UVB radiation occurs between 10 a.m. and 4 p.m. when the sun is highest in the sky and we are more likely to expose our skin on the beach or in the backyard. We are also literally closest to the sun, due to the tilt of the Earth's axis, meaning UVB has less distance to travel to reach our skin.

UVB exposure is greater at high altitudes than at sea level. This is because the atmosphere is thinner there, so there is less of its filtering effect between the sun and our skin. For example, at an altitude of 2000 metres, we are exposed to a third more UVB than at sea level. UVB also bounces off reflective surfaces like ice and snow, giving us a double hit. Along with the low humidity in really cold places, this is why the faces of mountaineers always look so weather-beaten.

UVB radiation should be greatest at the equator because the earth is a globe and the equator is closest to the sun. UVB from the sun has farther to go to reach the higher latitudes north or south of the equator. This has changed over the last century, as depletion of the ozone layer by greenhouse gases and chemicals like chloro-fluorocarbons means that more UVB is now able to get through, even at higher latitudes, in areas that used to be well protected by a thick effective ozone layer.

SUNLIGHT CAUSES DAMAGE TO SKIN CELLS

All solar radiation affects our skin and its functions in some way. It is progressively damaging to our skin chiefly because some skin components are able to absorb the energy in sunlight, and this process generates reactive oxygen molecules, which are known as free radicals. These reactive oxygen molecules then do what their name suggests: they react, almost immediately, with anything in the skin nearby. This wreaks havoc with the skin's function. In much the same way that rust progressively damages a metal object, the more sun we get, the more our skin and its structures becomes damaged. At the same time, damage caused by sunlight also sets off an inflammatory response, which contributes to the breakdown of collagen. The cumulative damage of prolonged exposure to the sun is called photoageing, and it can make us look prematurely old.

The early signs of sun damage are often difficult to see in the mirror. We can look at old photos and compare them to more recent ones, but it is often hard to be objective about our own appearance. One common way to check up on what is really going on involves taking pictures of the skin under UVA light (also known as a Wood's Lamp) as it can detect barely visible changes in the pigments in our skin. This kind of check-up can show the accumulated sun exposure relative to our age. Repeated examinations can also show how well a treatment program is working in reversing sun damage on the skin.

THE SUN'S EFFECT ON DIFFERENT SKIN TYPES

In practical terms, it is easiest to categorise skin into six different types, ranging from extremely fair (type 1) to very dark (type 6). This is the so-called Fitzpatrick Scale. The cumulative effects of regular sun exposure can be seen in all skin types, but they are more obvious and severe in people with type 1 skin, who burn more readily, don't tan easily and have a higher rate of skin cancers.

This is because fair skin has lower levels of melanin. Melanin is a chemical made by the skin that protects it against solar damage. Basically, melanin preferentially absorbs solar radiation, meaning it takes the bullet so other parts of the skin are spared. About five times less UVB enters dark skin when compared to light skin. This is chiefly due to more melanin.

Exposure to UV radiation also triggers the skin to make more melanin in order to protect the skin from getting too much sun in the future. We call this a tan, as our skin looks darker. This increased production of melanin can persist for several weeks after getting out in the sun, so our tan also persists for a while to protect us.

Melanin is not the only defence we have against sunlight. Healthy skin is naturally rich in antioxidants and efficient skin turnover also helps prevent any damage from remaining in the skin. Diets naturally high in antioxidants offer some protection against sun damage, mostly through reducing oxidative damage and dulling inflammation. However, anything that interferes with our skin's defences, like smoking, a poor diet or stress can make it easier for sunlight to do its damaging thing.

People who have other skin problems such as dermatitis must avoid too much exposure to the sun, as their condition means that their skin's defences are down. It is also important to remember that many cosmetic procedures affect our skin's ability to cope with sunlight, especially resurfacing procedures that temporarily reduce the thickness of the epidermis. This can allow more sunlight to get into the skin, and to get in deeper than normal. As detailed later in the treatment sections (Sections 7, 8, 9 and 10), protection from the sun is very important for anyone having or considering a cosmetic procedure.

LIMIT SUN EXPOSURE

There are many practical everyday steps to prevent excessive sun exposure and keep our skin looking and feeling younger for longer.

TIPS TO MINIMISE SUN DAMAGE TO YOUR SKIN

TIP	RATIONALE
Reduce or avoid unprotected exposure of our skin to sunlight.	Especially during peak hours for UVB radiation (generally between 10 a.m. and 4 p.m. in summer).
Seek out the shade.	A shady tree, gazebo or umbrella can reduce solar radiation reaching our skin by as much as 95 percent.
Don't be fooled by a cloudy day into thinking that you don't need to worry about the sun.	Clouds only modestly reduce the intensity of harmful UVB rays and have little effect on UVA. The weather service in summer often reports the UV index. It's always greatest on clear blue-sky days, but even on cloudy days in summer, it can still be high.
Don't be fooled by a cold day.	UV radiation is not related to temperature. On hot sunny days it's easy to remember to cover our skin, but all too often on cooler days we forget and our skin carries the burden.
Exposure to sunlight isn't limited to the outdoors.	We spend a lot of our working hours behind glass windows in the workplace or behind the wheel of a car. Glass blocks the transmission of UVB but not UVA. Most front windscreens are now treated to block some UVA, but side windows are often a problem. For example, the frequency of skin cancers is reported to be higher on the right side of the face in Australia and the left side in the USA. This is thought to be due to sunlight coming through the respective driver's side window.
Use physical barriers to sun exposure, including a wide-brimmed hat.	A good wide-brimmed hat will provide the equivalent of sun protection factor 7 for the nose, 3 for cheeks, 5 for neck and 2 for the chin.

TIP	RATIONALE
Sunglasses can help prevent wrinkles and sagging.	A wraparound style or a pair with side shields offers most protection. Remember, expensive brands do not always guarantee good UVA protection. Check the protection value of even cheap pairs to find the best option.
The right clothes will also help protect your skin from the sun.	All types of fabrics will disrupt the radiation of UV rays to a certain extent. A typical cotton shirt provides an Ultraviolet Protection Factor (UPF) – analogous to the sun protection factor (SPF) used to rate sunscreens – of less than 10. Tightly woven fibres, thick fabrics, wool and polyester materials are considerably higher. Dark coloured fabrics also have greater UPF than light coloured fabrics, but have the disadvantage of getting hot in the sun. It is now possible to buy clothing with a high UPF (15–50) that still retain a light, comfortable feel in summer. This is also very important when swimming as getting fabric wet halves its UPF.
Avoid sun lamps and tanning lounges.	These should not come near your precious skin – they pose a major risk of cancer.

SELECTING SUNSCREEN

The best sunscreen is the one we always put on before we go into the sun for extended periods. If it feels too greasy or sticky, smells unpleasant or looks bad on our skin, we won't ever use it. Even if it is the best sunscreen in the world, it is useless if its stays in the drawer. Just like we try out cosmetics, it is useful to try out the feel of different kinds of sunscreen before buying.

Another important consideration is the Sun Protection Factor (SPF). The SPF is a measure of how well a sunscreen prevents the skin from going red when exposed to UVB, and is the most important 'ingredient' when choosing protection to prevent photoageing. The best protection is achieved by a broad-spectrum, water resistant sunscreen with an SPF of 30+. A sunscreen with an SPF of 30+ will provide greater than 96 percent protection against UVB. However, a high SPF refers only to its actions on UVB, so doesn't necessarily mean total prevention of sun damage.

There is currently no good standard of protection from UVA and infrared rays. The best option is to look for products that have effective blockade across a broad spectrum, or at the very least care enough about UVA to put data on the label. For example, products that contain metal oxides (like zinc oxide and titanium dioxide) are usually very efficient sun blocks, reflecting and scattering light across most wavelengths, including UVA. Another ingredient to look for on the label is avobenzone, which offers good UVA protection.

SUNSCREEN TIPS

When looking to purchase sunscreen consider the following:

> To be effective, sunscreens should be reapplied every few hours while exposed to the sun, and after swimming or vigorous exercise, due to perspiration and/ or towel drying. The amount of sunscreen applied to the skin also makes a difference. Most of us use less than half the amount that was used to determine the SPF. To get the full effect you need to really slather it on. Alternatively, reapply the sun cream every 30 minutes or so to get cumulative protection.

> Sunscreens can be categorised as organic or inorganic. This has nothing to do with them being chemical and pesticide free, as with food labelling. Organic sunscreens use chemicals that absorb ultraviolet radiation, so preventing it from reaching into your skin. Inorganic sunscreens work by creating a thick coating of metal oxide particles to absorb, scatter and reflect UV radiation. Both work well, and can have comparable SPF factors; they just achieve it in different ways.

> Recent attention has been given to the presence of so-called 'nano-particles' in sun-creams and their supposed ability to penetrate into the skin rather than just sit on top of it. At present, however, there is insufficient data about either their effectiveness or their potential risks.

> Since oxidative stress is one of the ways sunlight causes skin damage and skin ageing, it is logical that antioxidants can prove useful in the defence against it. This is why many sun creams will also contain antioxidants. The role of antioxidants in skincare is discussed in chapter 9.

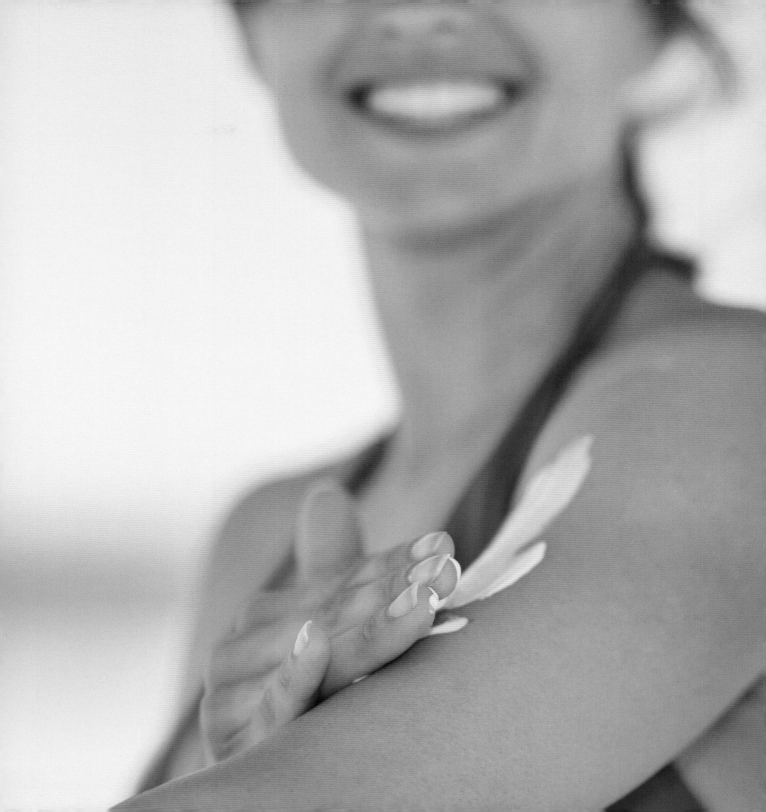

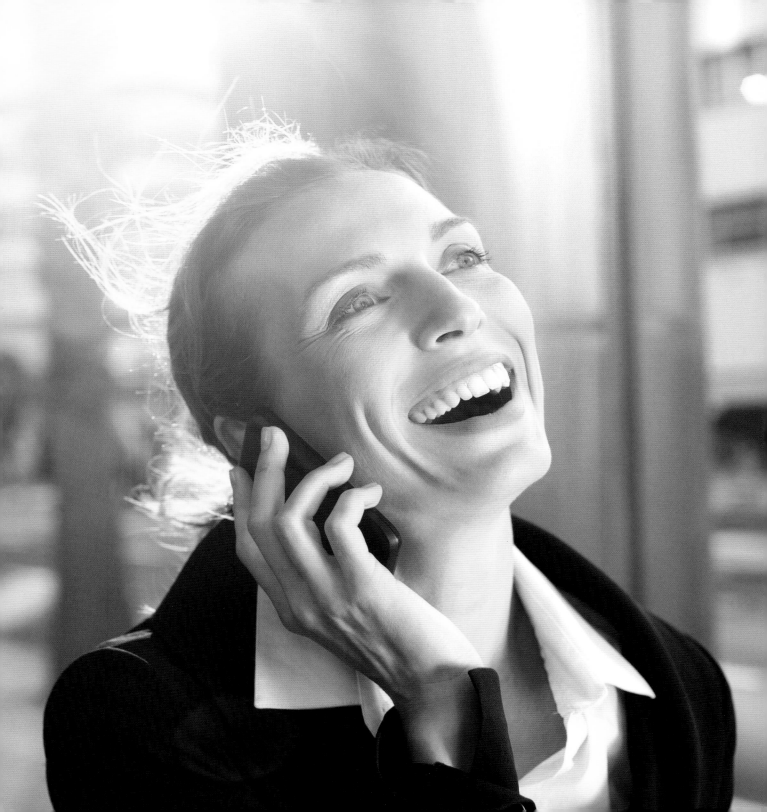

CHAPTER 07

SMOKE AND AIR POLLUTION

The air is filled with particles such as dust, pollen, soot, smoke and numerous droplets of various liquids. Each has the potential to land on our skin and influence its appearance. This is most graphically illustrated by the wrinkled face, prominent cheekbones and grey, dry skin of a heavy smoker. Even limited exposure makes a difference. For example, if we look at the faces of identical twins, which should be identical in every way as they were when they were young, the twin who has smoked (or smoked for a longer period of time) always looks older. It doesn't take much. Even the difference of a few extra years of smoking can be seen on the face. But it is not just cigarettes that have an influence; the closer to a busy road we live and work, for instance, the faster our skin appears to age.

SMOKE AND POLLUTION DAMAGES THE SKIN

Tobacco smoke is a mix of toxic chemicals, the most damaging of which are free radicals. These have a direct effect on your skin's surface as well as being transferred through the lungs and into the circulation to reach the skin from the inside. Free radicals in smoke cause a number of molecular changes to impair healing and healthy skin turnover. The skin's natural antioxidant defences are also so depleted.

The most well-known signs of smoking are wrinkles and lines on the face. These are typically on the mid to lower face (i.e. below the eyes, across the cheeks and on the jaw line). Pursing of the lips when inhaling and squinting when smoke gets in the eyes also contributes to the formation of 'crow's feet' wrinkles around the mouth and eyes. You don't even need to be the one inhaling for smoke to be a problem for your skin. Being near someone else's cigarette smoke is enough to cause the breakdown of matrix connective tissue and a disorganised healing response.

Smoking causes similar changes in the skin to those caused be the sun. Sun damage makes the effects of smoking much worse, and vice versa. Whether influenced by sun or smoke, excess wrinkles are the result of the same process: the connective tissue that holds young skin taut is broken down and inefficiently repaired. Even if you can't change your age, you can certainly reduce your exposure to sunlight and cigarette smoke.

Another result of smoking is a certain gauntness of the facial features. The skin becomes increasingly slack and is dragged downward by the wrinkles in the lower face, meaning on the upper part of the face the underlying bony contours become more prominent. The skin also takes on a grey appearance. This is thought to be the result of reduced blood flow to the skin (which itself contributes to impaired healing).

Just as with cigarette smoke, it is thought that airborne toxins contained in pollution are able to penetrate the skin and generate free radicals. Some airborne particles can act as carriers for toxic chemicals and heavy metals. Some environmental pollutants also increase the sensitivity of skin to sunlight and can mean free radicals are generated when the polluted skin is exposed to sunlight. This enhances the damage to the skin caused by sun exposure and further accelerates skin ageing.

One particular toxin gaining attention in skin ageing is ozone. In the Earth's atmosphere, ozone acts to protect you against the harmful effects of sunlight, but ground level or 'bad' ozone dissolves into the oils of our skin and depletes its natural antioxidants, triggering inflammation and matrix remodelling. Bad ozone is created by emissions from industrial facilities and vehicle exhaust when it reacts with sunlight, especially during the summer when ground ozone levels are at their highest.

PREVENTING SMOKE FROM DAMAGING THE SKIN

Quit and stay smoke free. There are lots of effective therapies that can help you to stop smoking. The good news is that quitting for good can reverse some of the skin damage caused by smoking.

The regular use of antioxidants can reduce the effects of free radicals caused by smoke and pollution, but they may not penetrate the skin particularly well. Nonetheless, they are ready and waiting to block any airborne radicals. Many cosmetic products contain antioxidants, including plant-derived polyphenols, flavonoids and vitamins. Remember that their effect is probably only partial at best if you continue to smoke.

Healthy skin forms an almost impenetrable barrier to the outside world, with layers of tightly packed dead cells and oils that are continuously shed and replaced. Healthy barrier functions are the best defence against smoke and other toxins. This is why it is important to preserve or enhance the barrier functions of the skin as we get older. This includes skincare regimens involving the use of humectants (Chapter 8), emollients and low-irritation cleansers, along with avoiding the application of products that can promote skin dryness. The more your skin can keep out the toxins, the less damage will be done and the slower your skin will age.

SMOKING AND COSMETIC TREATMENTS

Reducing the effects of previous smoking is one the most common reasons for having cosmetic procedures performed. Smokers have more skin problems and may be in greater need of cosmetic treatments at a younger age than non-smokers. Smoking interferes with wound healing, so the response to treatment with procedures that stimulate collagen synthesis – like volumisers, fibroblasts, peels and laser – is reduced if you still smoke. At the same time the risk of complications is increased. Indeed, some practitioners will not start a treatment program until their clients have been smoke-free for six months or more. Although it may be harder, giving up smoking is a far better investment than any cosmetic procedure.

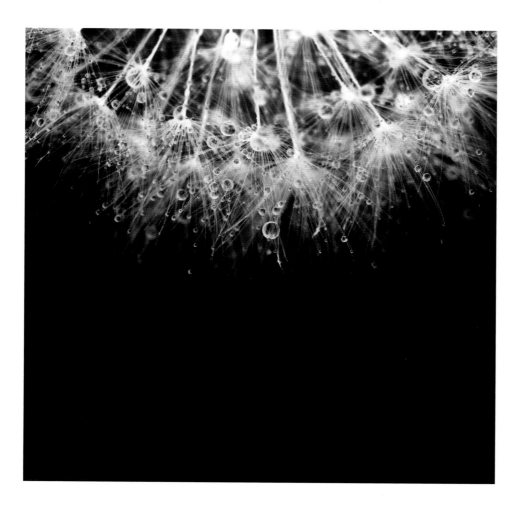

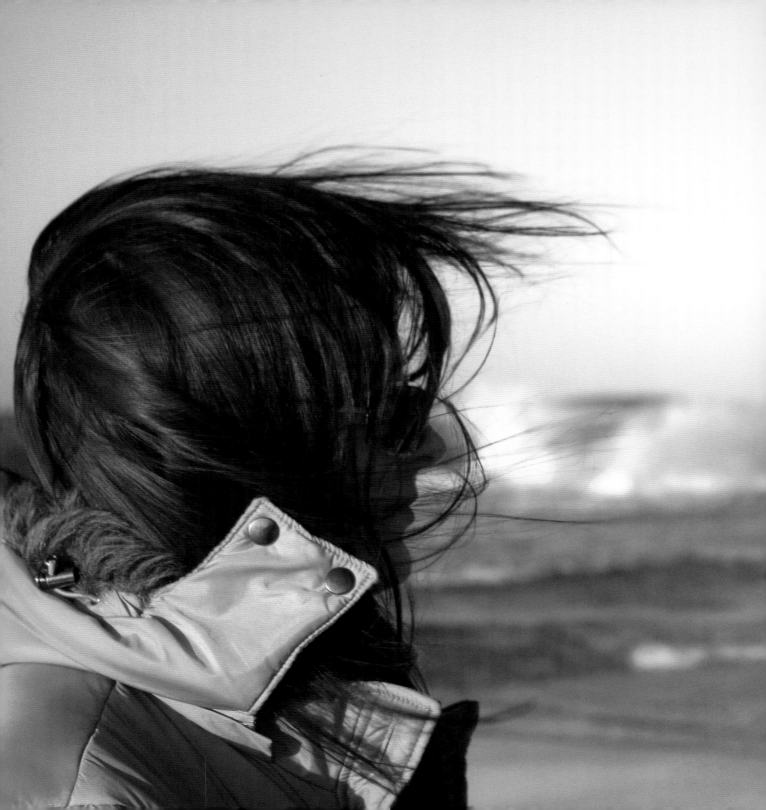

CHAPTER 08:

OTHER ENVIRONMENTAL IMPACTS ON AGEING SKIN

There are a surprising number of sources of skin damage that are often overlooked. These include excess humidity, wind, gravity and some of the components of water.

HUMIDITY AND AGEING SKIN

Humidity is the amount of water vapour in the air. These water droplets are invisible to the naked eye, but make a real difference to the appearance of our skin. In a dry environment, the skin loses some of its moisture. This makes the surface of the skin look rough, as fine lines and wrinkles become more visible, especially on the face. Skin drying can also trigger inflammation, a negative factor in skin ageing. Although these changes are largely reversible in the short term, the cumulative effects of long-term exposure to low humidity may persist in our skin.

Dry air or low humidity is not just experienced in dry climates. In winter, the heating of cold outdoor air can decrease indoor humidity levels, wherever you live, to below 30 percent, which is not much different from the level found in the Sahara Desert. This is one reason why many people suffer from dry itchy skin in the colder months (known as winter-itch) especially as they get older.

Another example is what happens to the skin during a flight, as the relative humidity in an aeroplane cabin typically drops to less than 10 percent. This is why many of us experience dry, sore eyes, fine wrinkles and dry, itchy skin even after relatively short flights.

These changes can be prevented. If you don't want dry wrinkled skin stepping off the plane, occlusive moisturisers can help to reduce moisture loss, while humectants can recover lost fluid.

The same goes for the office every day, where air conditioning can reduce humidity. The importance of moisturising is discussed in chapter 18. (Another simple solution is to use a humidifier in your office. This can help keep moisture in your skin. Set it between 45 percent and 60 percent.)

The average temperature of your skin is mostly determined by how hot it is outside. The hotter it gets, the hotter your skin gets. On a warm day as the temperature goes up, blood flow to the skin increases. This makes you look more flushed and serves to dissipate unwanted heat. As we get older, the skin is less effective at moving blood around, so we are more vulnerable to overheating.

Moisture loss from the skin also increases in hot temperatures. This is not just the evaporative cooling effect of extra perspiration on hot days. The same drying and wrinkling effects on the skin that occur in an air-conditioned aeroplane also occur when your skin gets hot. If it is both hot and dry, the effects on your skin are even more pronounced.

WIND AND AGEING SKIN

Your skin is also exposed to the force of wind, which can increase the evaporation of moisture from the skin. On hot days this is a good thing in that sweating helps to keep you cool, but it also means the skin is left drier. On cold days, wind is chilling and can chap the skin. Hot or cold, a day out in the wind can also make your skin itchy, wrinkled and dry for the same water-loss reasons that a plane trip or a day in the desert does.

Often, as wind makes the day feel cooler, we may not take the same protections from the sun for our skin as we would on a hot, still day, which can leave the skin exposed to solar damage. However, some people think that drying of the skin may make sunburn more likely. In fact, we generally treat a face that has been reddened by the sun with moisturisers and the redness goes away, which suggests that the moisture content of the skin, and its decline on a windswept day, does play a role.

GRAVITY AND AGEING SKIN

With gravity weighing on us all of the time, it's hardly a surprise that our skin sags downwards rather than up. Gravity is a force of nature that contributes to the weathering of our skin. Whether we are talking about a longer nose or earlobes, drooping jowls or breasts, gravity plays a role. (It is not all downhill, however, because as we get older our eyebrows generally move upward, pulled up by the altogether greater force of our forehead wrinkles!)

Because the effects of gravity on our skin are so obvious, the fight against them has extended into the cosmetic realm. Some practitioners recommend activities like regularly standing on our head (known as sirsasana in yoga) or being tilted head-down for periods of time to give a 'natural face lift'. This can be a great yoga technique and some women find it relaxing; however, there is no definitive evidence that it fixes wrinkles.

Another common gravity-defying recommendation is to massage our skin every day in the opposite direction of gravity. Unfortunately, there is no evidence that this works.

BATHING AND IMMERSION

Our skin is not just exposed to the air. We also often immerse it in water, when we wash or swim.

Chlorination is the most common way that swimming pools are kept free of bugs; however, swimming in chlorinated water has a drying effect on our skin. It also generates by-products that can be irritating to the skin. This is why your skin can feel chalky after being in the pool. That's not to say you should give up swimming, as it is excellent for health and fitness. Instead, try using a water-stable emollient before your swim to help keep your skin moist. It's also useful to take a brief shower afterwards and thoroughly rinse your skin with fresh water. Don't use the soap provided by the pool, which often makes things worse. Pat yourself dry and follow with an occlusive moisturiser.

Ozone is a strong oxidiser, capable of adversely affecting the integrity of the skin. While many modern pools now use electrically generated ozone instead of chlorine to kill bugs in the water, it can be problematic in terms of skin health.

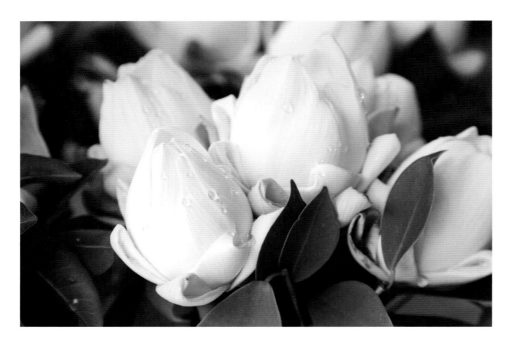

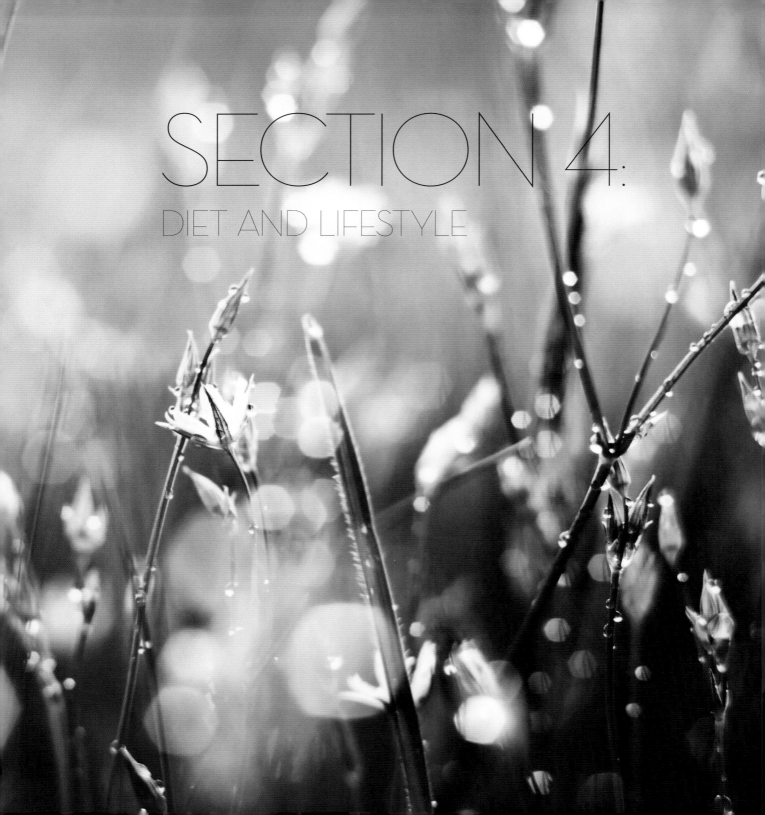

SECTION 4:
DIET AND LIFESTYLE

Health starts from within and unless you are prepared to battle ageing from within, then you'll never be totally happy with the results of any interventions in the longer term. Let food be your medicine and your skin will be a key beneficiary. There are foods to avoid as well as foods to harness for their healing properties. Sugar is one of the main culprits when it comes to accelerating skin ageing. Sugar is your enemy and if you can do one thing to stop the ravages of ageing, then give up sugar!

The link between exercise and good skin is less well known. We do know that regular exercise is a key tool in any anti-ageing program. Exercise promotes healthy circulation and this will help with skin health. Blood carries oxygen and nutrients into all cells of the body, including the skin. It also carries toxins out of the body, and the skin benefits from this function as well.

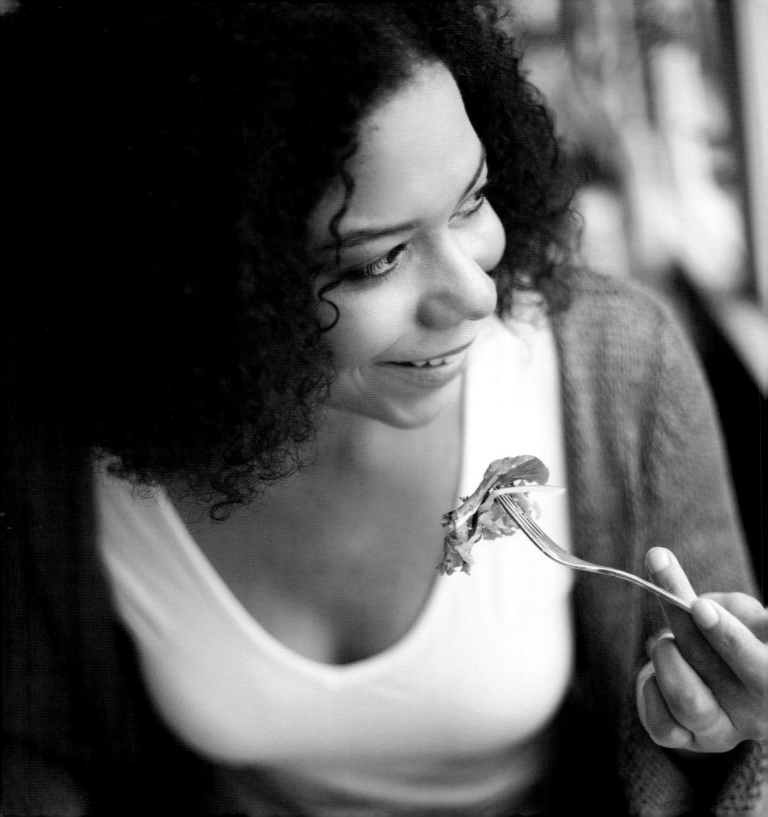

CHAPTER 09

ANTIOXIDANTS

Everything that damages your skin, from sunlight and smoking to stress or lack of sleep, does so partly by generating highly reactive and toxic by-products of oxygen in your skin. Normally, oxygen molecules have an even number of electrons, but when something (such as cigarette smoke or ultraviolet light) consumes or removes one of the electrons from the molecule it is left with an unpaired (free) electron. These are known as free radicals. This free electron makes oxygen highly reactive, hence the alternative name for free radicals, Reactive Oxygen Species (or ROS for short).

To fix this imbalance, free radicals regain their missing electron by stealing it from other chemicals. In fact, they can quickly react with almost anything they come in contact with, including DNA, lipids in cell membranes, proteins and other vital structures, leaving them damaged. Damage caused by free radicals (known as oxidative damage or injury) is a key trigger for inflammation and matrix breakdown in the skin – both are significant processes in skin ageing.

Antioxidants are a common form of defence against free radicals and are incorporated into skincare products as 'cosmeceuticals' and available as dietary supplements as 'nutraceuticals'. However, the clinical efficacy of these plant-derived compounds and vitamins is not well understood.

The skin has its own antioxidant defence systems, the job of which is to remove free radicals before they can do damage. These defences include enzymes that directly catalyse the destruction of free radicals, as well as antioxidant 'decoys' that prevent damage by 'taking the bullet' themselves, thereby preventing other more important elements of your skin from becoming attacked and damaged by the free radicals. In this category are the key vitamin antioxidants, vitamin E and vitamin C.

If the production of toxic free radicals outstrips your antioxidant defence mechanisms, a state of oxidative stress occurs. This is one of the most important causes of ageing in the skin. There is good evidence that the effectiveness of these antioxidant defences correlates with the health of the skin and its appearance. In general, the body's production of antioxidants declines as you grow older, while the production of and cumulative exposure to free radicals increases, overwhelming the skin's defences and leading to oxidative stress and as well as to ageing itself.

In this context, it makes perfect sense to target free radicals as a means to slow ageing. Almost all anti-ageing strategies over the past forty years have included antioxidants as a central ingredient. At least one in five women regularly takes antioxidant supplements. Although the idea of antioxidants is sound, the long-term beneficial effects on the health and appearance of the skin are yet to be understood. Diets naturally high in antioxidants are associated with better health and so may well impact upon the skin, but few clinical trials have made a direct connection between antioxidant supplements and smoother skin.

VITAMIN E (TOCOPHEROL)

Vitamin E is perhaps the most important antioxidant naturally present in human skin. It acts as a decoy target for free radicals, which modify it instead of attacking something more important. It is then regenerated by vitamin C, allowing it to do its job over and over again, neutralising free radicals and protecting our skin from damage. As an oil- and fat-soluble antioxidant it is particularly effective in preventing free radical damage to lipids in the cell membranes. In addition, vitamin E also has significant positive effects on inflammation and immune function.

Vitamin E is not made by the skin but rather, it must be obtained from our diet. A standard daily Western diet contains three or four milligrams of vitamin E. This is less than half the recommended daily intake and even less than the optimal intake.

VITAMIN C (ASCORBATE, ASCORBIC ACID)

Vitamin C (also known as ascorbate) is the most plentiful natural antioxidant in our skin (and has some natural benefits for us in terms of sun protection). Like vitamin E, it functions as a decoy target for free radicals. In addition, vitamin C regenerates vitamin E and is a necessary co-factor in collagen synthesis. Vitamin C is rapidly depleted in the skin by sunlight and smoking.

We can get all our vitamin C for normal physiological needs from our diet, but not for maximum UV protection of the skin, so we need to use products that contain vitamin C. Topical vitamin C can increase dermal vitamin C levels by up to 20 times the natural level.

VITAMIN A AND BETA-CAROTENE

Vitamin A is a member of the retinoid family (chapter 20) of chemicals that have potent effects on ageing skin. In fact, retinoids are the only topical agents for which there are numerous large double blind studies in ageing and sun-damaged skin.

VITAMIN B3 (NIACIN)

Vitamin B3 (niacin) is a family of antioxidant compounds that are essential to the body for energy metabolism and DNA repair.

MAGNESIUM

Magnesium is one of the most important nutrients that our body needs. It is a macro-mineral that contributes to maintaining the strength and tautness of the skin, and promoting skin health by, for example, helping combat free radicals.

ALPHA-LIPOIC ACID

Alpha-lipoic acid is a free radical scavenger that protects the skin, and has additional benefits in regenerating the skin's antioxidant defences.

COENZYME Q10

Most free radicals are generated as oxygen shuttles in and out of the mitochondria, structures that provide the energy in every cell. This means that the mitochondria are also the major target for oxidative damage. If we damage our mitochondria, this means less efficient use of oxygen for energy production along with a further increase in free radical production – a vicious cycle common to many ageing processes.

Coenzyme Q10 (CoQ10) is a key antioxidant inside the mitochondria as well as an important component of efficient energy production. Reduced levels of CoQ10 leads to increased formation of free radicals. The levels of CoQ10 in the skin decline from our mid-thirties onwards. This decline is fastest in those who repeatedly expose their skin to sun and in smokers. Because of this association, it makes sense to bolster our CoQ10 levels and its defence against free radical attack.

CoQ10 is synthesised in the human body with the assistance of numerous vitamins, including vitamin B, vitamin C and folic acid. Of these, vitamin B6 (also known as pyridoxine) probably has the biggest impact.

One way to maintain CoQ10 levels is to ensure an adequate intake of pyridoxine, which is found in meat, poultry, fish, wholegrain products, vegetables, beans and nuts. Too much alcohol or coffee may deplete our vitamin B6 levels.

RESVERATROL

Resveratrol is part of a group of plant compounds called polyphenols. They can have an antioxidant effect in the body, and may be beneficial in terms of protecting the skin against photoageing caused by sun exposure.

MELATONIN

Melatonin is a hormone produced naturally in the human body. Its job in regulating sleep cycles is well known and is now widely used in the prevention and treatment of jet-lag.

FOOD SOURCES CONTAINING ANTIOXIDANTS
> Vitamin E is found in leafy green vegetables, nuts and seeds, whole grains, corn, soy, and some meats, dairy products and vegetable oils. However, many of the vegetable oils sold in supermarkets have had the vitamin E removed during processing, so always check the label. Some products are now fortified with extra vitamin E.
> Vitamin C is commonly associated with citrus fruits like oranges and lemons, but vitamin C levels are even higher in rosehip and rose petals, and in berries and currants. Vitamin C is also found in green leafy vegetables, brassicas and capsicum. It is widely used as a food preservative, especially in processed juices.
> Vitamin A is found in both plant and animal products. In plants, it is present in richly coloured carotenoids, such as beta-carotene, which is converted into vitamin A during digestion. Brightly coloured plants are a good place to get vitamin A from and include carrots, broccoli, kale, sweet potato, spinach, pumpkin, romaine lettuce, capsicum tomatoes, carrots, strawberries, mango, apricots, rockmelon and watermelon. Vitamin A is also found in naturally high amounts in liver, beef, pork, chicken, turkey, fish, eggs and butter. Fresh is best, as vitamin A can be depleted from foods during preparation, cooking, or storage (free radicals are produced during prolonged storage or when the food is exposed to high temperatures).
> Niacin is widely found in a healthy, balanced diet, including in meat, grains, dairy, fruit and vegetables.
> Foods rich in selenium include meat, tuna and eggs. Plants grown in selenium-rich soils also contain increased levels of selenium, including wheat germ, nuts (particularly Brazil nuts), oats, whole-wheat bread, bran, brown rice, turnips, garlic and barley.
> Foods rich in alpha-lipoic acid include potatoes, carrots, broccoli, beets and yams, as well as red meat.
> CoQ10 containing foods with the highest level are those containing the largest numbers of mitochondria, such as liver, kidney and heart, fish and whole grains.
> Melatonin levels are high in medicinal plants including St. John's wort and feverfew. It is also found in bananas, tomatoes, apples and Montmorency cherries, as well as oats, sweet corn, ginger and rice bran. The seeds of white and black mustard, wolfberry and fenugreek, in particular, also contain high levels of melatonin.

CARNOSINE

Carnosine is a multifunctional antioxidant found in meat, and as such is one antioxidant often lacking in a vegetarian diet. Its long-term effects on human ageing are unclear, although it is widely touted as an effective anti-ageing therapy.

POLYPHENOLS

Polyphenols are a large family of naturally occurring plant-derived antioxidants. Most polyphenols are flavonoids (also known as tannins because they give plants their flavour and colour), but as all flavonoids are polyphenols, these names are often used interchangeably. Some of the most popular polyphenols used as nutraceuticals include:

> **Astaxanthin.** A pink carotenoid found in high concentrations in salmon and shrimp.
> **Epigallocatechin gallate (EGCG).** Found in green tea.
> **Silymarin and silybin.** Found in milk thistle.
> **Quercitin.** Found in onions, apples, green tea and black tea.
> **Hesperidin and rutin.** Found in citrus fruits.
> **Proanthocyanidin.** Found in grape seed extract.
> **Genistein, daidzein, aglycone and other isoflavones.** Found in soybean products.
> **Resveratrol.** Found in grapes, wine, peanuts and knotweed.
> **Ellagic acid.** Found in many red fruits and berries, including raspberries, strawberries, blackberries, cranberries, grapes and pomegranate, as well as and some nuts, including pecans and walnuts.
> **Sulphoraphane and indole-3-carbinol.** Found in broccoli as well as other cruciferous vegetables (members of the cabbage family).
> **Lycopene.** Found in red and pink fruits such as tomatoes, watermelon, pink grapefruit, pink guava, papaya and rosehip.
> **Lutein.** Found in green leafy vegetable like spinach, kale, collard greens, romaine lettuce, as well as in leeks, peas and egg yolks.
> **Luteolin.** Found in herbs and vegetables including parsley, olive oil, basil, peppermint, capsicum, rosemary and celery.
> **Hydroxytyrosol.** Found in olive juice and oil.
> **Curcumin.** Derived from turmeric.
> **Ginkgo flavonglycosides.** The extract of Ginkgo leaves.

> **Caffeic acid, caffeic acid phenethyl ester (CAPE) and ferulic acid.** Found in many plants, but is particularly high in coffee berry (the unripe coffee bean), apple and orange seeds, peanuts, artichoke, pineapple, cooked sweet corn as well as the bran of rice, rye, wheat, oats, barley and flax. CAPE is also high in bee propolis (which is carried back from pine sap by honey bees).

Many products don't contain just one polyphenol but provide multiple extracts from things like green tea, pomegranate, grapes and rosehip. Each of these compounds, extracts and many others have been shown to reduce free radical damage in a laboratory setting, but how well they work in the human body is hotly debated. Evidence of any significant effect is weak at best. In the last few years the American FDA have removed the popular Oxygen Radical Absorbance Capacity (ORAC) Database, which ranked foods according to their antioxidant content, arguing that "no evidence shows the beneficial effects of polyphenol-rich foods can be attributed to the antioxidant properties of these foods, and data for antioxidant capacity generated (in test tube experiments) cannot be extrapolated to real life effects".

HOW DO WE GET MORE ANTIOXIDANTS?

The best way to ensure a diet that is high in antioxidants and good for our skin is to remember the SLOW foods acronym: Slow foods are those that are Seasonal, Local, Organic and Whole.

A diet high in fresh produce is always best. It is the nutrients in fresh food that convey the most health-giving properties. Consequently, the greatest benefits can be achieved when those nutrients are at their highest, meaning when foods are in season and when they are at their freshest. The more transportation, handling, storage and processing involved in getting food to your table, the lower the nutrient levels of the food are likely to be. Where possible, buy local produce. Imported food may look peachy, but it has probably been on the road a lot longer than local food. Nutrient losses occur with every freeze and thaw cycle (transported in the back of our car, leaving the packet out, etc.) and even more nutrients are lost during cooking. Buy fresh only if it can be eaten within the next few days. Putting it in the fridge slows the degradation process, but does not stop it. Fruit and veggies should be stored in different areas of the fridge because ripe fruit releases chemicals that cause some veggies to lose their nutrients.

The best way to buy and store fruit and vegetables is whole. Buying cut fruit and vegetables may seem an easier option, but is only beneficial if you are ready to eat them immediately. Cutting them up and exposing their contents to light results in the loss of nutritional properties. The less processed a food is, the higher the antioxidant potential. Eat whole fruit over fruit juice, every time.

The most common cereals we see in our diet are heavily refined, meaning that the bran and germ (which contain most of the good bits such as antioxidants and soluble fibre) have been removed and only the inner starchy part of the grain remains. So choose whole grain foods, which retain either intact, flaked or broken grain kernels. Try a breakfast cereal that includes whole grain, not just wheat. Switch white bread with whole grain bread, or bread that is high in whole rye, barley, sunflower, linseed (flaxseed) or bulgur. And consider oat bran rather than just oats, as brans are more concentrated and therefore we need to eat less to gain the same nutritional benefit.

Most of us get into the habit of eating the same foods week in, week out, but it pays to choose something different from time to time. Don't let your diet (or your food) go stale! It is often said we should all aim to have at least five serves of fruit and vegetables per day, but this shouldn't be the same stuff all the time. Follow the seasons to get the freshest produce at the right time of the year. It does not need to be expensive or exotic to be healthy, but it has to be enjoyable for us to keep eating it regularly.

Food is one of life's great pleasures, so when we are eating, why not make the most of a great opportunity? Fruits and vegetables, whole grains, legumes, nuts and seeds give us more for each spoonful (and generally fewer calories) than processed food – and they taste better too. But it is not just plants. Lean meat is more nutrient-dense than fatty mince. These foods give us more nutritional return for every calorie, so it makes sense to eat them for our general health as well as the health of our skin.

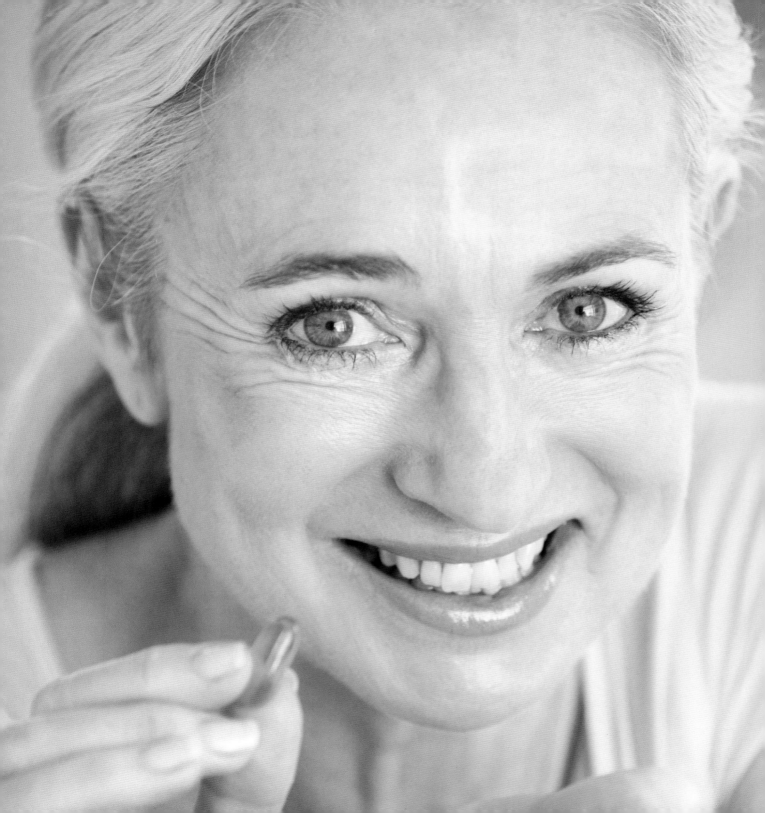

CHAPTER 10
FAT AND THE
AGEING PROCESS

One of the most important changes that occurs as we get older is an increase in the amount of fat in our bodies. Most of us will go up a dress size about every five years of our adult life. At least every second adult will become obese in his or her lifetime. This has major implications for our health. Controlling our waistline is the most important health issue we will probably face, as being overweight is responsible for up to 70 percent of chronic disease, increasing the risks of conditions such as diabetes, heart disease and certain cancers. Being overweight also affects the health of our skin and its appearance.

Gaining weight obviously stretches the skin. This can lead to stretch marks (also known as striae), which are most commonly found on the stomach, thighs, hips, buttocks and breasts. Striae are caused by damage to the connective tissue fibres of the dermis. Subsequent scarring realigns new connective tissue perpendicular to the direction of greatest tension. This creates smooth bands of thinner-looking skin, or stretch marks.

This is a particular problem for yo-yo dieters, women who lose lots of weight then put it back on again, and then try to lose it again, only to put it on again. There is some evidence that repeatedly losing and gaining weight stretches the skin irreversibly, especially on the face. This can contribute to sagging and facial lines.

AGEING AND CELLULITE

Another obvious change as we age is the more prominent appearance of cellulite, the unsightly 'cottage cheese' dimpling of the skin found mostly over the fat-rich thighs, buttocks and hips. It occurs in almost all women to a greater or lesser extent, but is more common as we get older, and particularity as we get fatter. Cellulite is caused by architectural changes in the boundary between the dermis and the underlying fat layer, which means some fat is irregularly squeezed up into the connective tissue between the two.

Another change in the skin in those who are overweight is the proliferation of soft pink skin tags (known as acrochordons). They are typically about the size of a grain of rice and found mostly around the neck, and in the armpits and groin, but they can sometimes occur on the face. They are not harmful or cancerous and do not grow or change. They do, however, sometimes get caught on clothing or necklaces, which can be irritating – and they are a reminder that something is out of balance.

WHY DO WE GET FAT?

Food provides energy in the form of calories. Some of this energy goes to fuel chemical reactions inside the body and provides the vital energy for every cell to do what needs to be done to keep the body functioning as it should. This is known as metabolism. Any excess energy is stored as fat, whether it was originally consumed as fat, carbohydrate or protein. If the energy supply exceeds our demands, our fat storage swells, particularly under the skin in the buttocks and breasts. Today, most people in the Western world eat more calories than required for their metabolism and daily energy expenditure through physical activity. Slowly but surely, they get fatter as they age. They are not always gluttonous or eating super-sized meals. They are just eating a little bit more than they burn, day after day. The average daily weight gain of most adults is the equivalent of no more than two extra mouthfuls of food, but over the decades it all adds up. There are many other factors that can also play a role in weight gain, including stress, the proliferation of processed foods, the addition of sugar to many food products, and increased demands by work causing a more sedentary lifestyle.

WEIGHT MANAGEMENT

This is one of the most important strategies to ensure our general health and that of our skin. If we create a negative energy balance by eating fewer calories and increasing our physical activity, our fat stores will go down. (But not all exercise is equal. As well as diet, weight resistance exercise plus aerobic exercise gives the greatest waist girth reduction, not aerobic exercise alone.)

Sometimes only minor changes are required to reduce the energy content of our diet and the fat under our skin. For example, the energy in a can of Coke® is around 500 kJ, so to lose the waist girth, subtracting the soft drink from your daily routine may be all that it takes to tip the balance.

It can be useful to regulate some or all food intake according to a plan. There are many diets out there. Each requires adherence to a formula, recipe book or strategy for success. The media is full of claims that one diet may be better than another, producing better weight loss or smoother glucose control because of a particular (magical) mix of nutrients. Rigorous studies of different diets have failed to show any clear winner. On average they all achieve about the same rate of weight loss. It is likely that the mere process of embracing dietary restrictions, and actively thinking about what we eat tends to help us eat less and eat better.

Diets that promote weight management can be broadly divided into four categories, although most share a number of common elements:

> Low-fat diets
> Low-carbohydrate diets (also known as high-protein diets)
> Low-calorie diets
> Low-GI diets

In essence, they all work by getting us to focus on just one aspect of our diet, and ignore everything else for the sake of simplicity. This makes each diet easy to understand and maintain. We can do it ourselves (e.g. by counting carbs or calories, or substituting low-fat foods for high-fat ones, and so on) or simply follow the recipe book or diet plan that makes these calculations for us.

Meal replacement programs are also sometimes used as an alternative to organising our own diet. This strategy of replacing certain meals is generally more successful than trying to limit calorie intake across all meals. This has made meal replacements some of the most popular of all commercial weight loss plans. However, their key limitation is the lack of flexibility, limited food choice and predictability. Many do not include an education component, so that when the program is completed we haven't learnt self-reliance with regard to our diet. Weight management needs to be a lifelong commitment, not a temporary fix. Ideally diets and meal replacements should be considered as a kick-start to a weight-loss program, which ultimately sees us take control of what we eat and maintain a healthy eating strategy throughout our life. Low-calorie, food-restrictive diets are not a long-term solution; we need to exercise moderation, not restriction. A healthy lifestyle that includes eating unprocessed foods (ones that are as close to their natural state as possible) and taking regular exercise is the way to go.

Successful weight management also involves changing how we eat as well as what we eat. In particular, it requires us to break old habits and form new ones. Simple tricks include using smaller plates, smaller utensils and serving smaller portions. Reducing snacks and comfort food as a source of unwanted calories is also important.

It can also be useful to keep a food diary of what we are eating. This can be in a book or an app. Studies have shown that dieters who kept a daily food diary lost more weight than those who didn't. Again it appears that the act of paying close attention to what we are eating, and recognising that our choices matter, is a key part of achieving and maintaining weight loss.

OMEGA-3: EATING MORE OF THE GOOD FAT

Some dietary fats are essential for good health and good skin. The most well-known of these are the omega-3 (ω-3) polyunsaturated fatty acids, which we know simply as omega-3s (or vitamin F). The body uses omega-3s to make chemicals (known as eicosanoids) that control a number of important pathways relevant to ageing – including inflammation, immune system function, oxidative stress and cell growth. A diet high in omega-3 fatty acids is associated with a lower risk of heart disease and some cancers, including those of the skin. A regular healthy intake of omega-3s is also associated with fewer wrinkles and slower skin ageing. It is unclear whether this is because omega-3s directly help the skin or because a high amount of omega-3 in our diet promotes general overall health.

There are many ways to get more omega-3s in our diet. It is commonly recommended that we should try to consume a meal of oily fish (such as salmon, herring, mackerel, anchovies, sardines and, to a lesser extent, tuna) two to three times every week. Oily fish is naturally high in the omega-3s, eicosapentaenoic acid (EPA) and docosahexaenoic acid (DHA). Although some people enjoy this fishy diet, many find that this is difficult to achieve because of cost, taste or smell.

We can also get omega-3s from plants, because most plants contain alpha linolenic acid (ALA) or stearidonic acid (STA), chemicals that can be converted to DHA in our body. STA is more easily converted, so it is more potent than ALA, however the conversion of either is partial at best. Some plants that contain high levels of ALA and STA include vegetable oils (like soya bean and canola oils), green leafy vegetables, flaxseed, purslane, sea buckthorn, chia seeds, algae, kiwifruit, lignon berries, raspberries, walnuts, lettuce and peas.

Because consumers want to get even more omega-3s without fish, a number of products – including bread, yoghurt, orange juice, pasta, milk, eggs, infant formula and even ice cream – can now come fortified with omega-3s.

You can also get omega-3s from supplements. The most common of these contain fish oil or krill oil. You have to take quite a lot of them to get a decent return (which can be expensive) and some people find them too fishy for their taste. Some fish oils may also contain toxic ocean pollutants, which are concentrated within the omega-3 acids. The environmental impact of catching fish or krill for oil should also be considered.

As an alternative, many women take concentrated ALA and STA supplements derived from plants, like flaxseed oil, oil of evening primrose, walnut oil, borage oil, hemp oil and even Echium oil (from Paterson's curse). You need to take more than with fish oil to get the same benefit, but there is much less of a fishy taste!

TOPICAL USE OF OMEGA-3

What if we put omega-3s directly onto our skin? Well, ALA and STA are already found in many cosmetic products, mostly in liposomes or nano-particles. Whether omega-3s actually work as a wrinkle cream is unclear. The big problem is that these fats can go off very easily, making them smell bad or change colour, so they would have a short shelf life or need to be kept in the fridge unless they are mixed with lots of antioxidants which prevent the fats from going off.

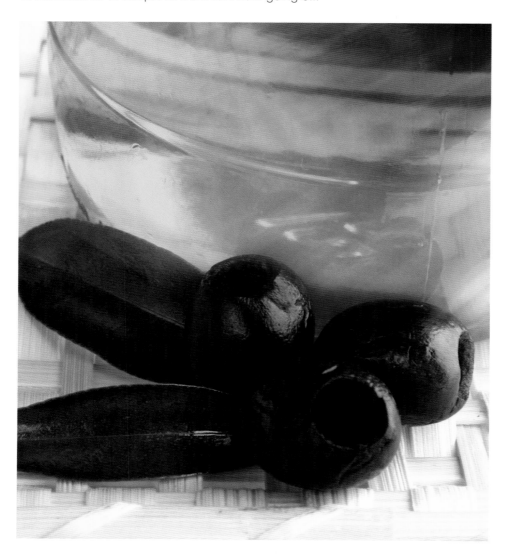

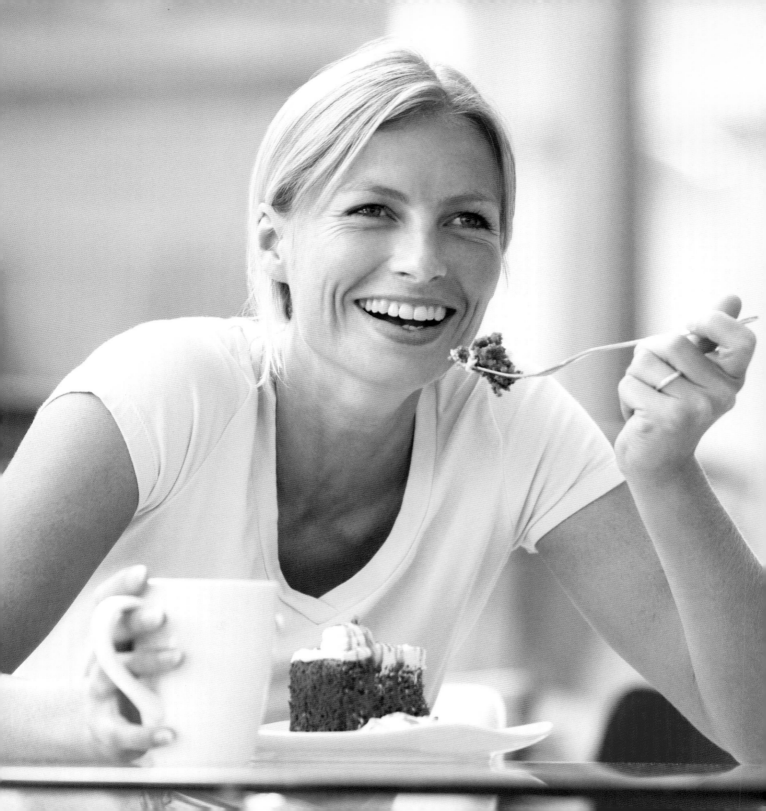

CHAPTER 11

SUGAR ACCELERATES THE AGEING PROCESS

During any cooking process, a chemical reaction occurs between sugars and proteins in the food. This is known as glycation or browning. This magical chemistry confers the colour, flavour and aromas of cooked foods, such as the crust on a loaf of bread. Because the human body also contains sugars and proteins, the same sort of chemistry is also possible inside us, and years of slow cooking at 37°C will eventually make all of us a little crusty.

ADVANCED GLYCATION END-PRODUCTS (AGES)

Over a lifetime, the amount and variety of glycation in our tissues slowly but progressively increases, at the rate of about four percent per year. The chemical products of these reactions are often known as AGEs (Advanced Glycation End-products).

After things become modified by AGEs they seldom work the same. For example, AGE modification of collagen in our skin leads to less efficient packing of fibres and the formation of inter-molecular cross-links, making the skin less flexible and less resilient to harm. Put simply, AGE-ing makes the skin age! AGEs also trigger an inflammatory response to attempt to rectify harm. Inflammation and disorganised healing are also major contributors to skin ageing.

Too much sugar accelerates the formation of AGEs in the skin. This is why people with diabetes have increased AGE levels in their skin, and hence older looking skin. Excessive sunlight exposure also increases AGE cross-linking in the skin. Cigarette smoke is high in AGEs and their reactive precursors, formed during the curing, browning and burning of tobacco leaves. Altogether, this is a recipe for getting older skin much sooner than we desire.

A number of widely available supplements have been reported to reduce the accumulation of AGEs, including benfotiamine, alpha-lipoic acid, carnosine, pyridoxine and rytine. Their effects appear modest at best, and they cannot eliminate AGEs that are already there, in much the same way that antioxidants don't work after the reactive oxygen species have finished reacting.

Some of the AGEs we accumulate in our body come from our diet. In particular, many of the highly processed foods we eat contain AGEs. This has a number of consequences. Browning effects produce flavours, textures and aromas that give many foods their appeal. For example, the crunch of crisps is achieved by cooking at very high temperature and low humidity. Sure the crisps taste better, not to mention that 'extra crunch', but at what cost? Often this processing will have negative effects on your skin.

RELATIONSHIP BETWEEN DIET AND AGES

There is a strong relationship between the levels of AGEs in our skin and the amount of AGEs consumed in our diets. It could be said that we are as old as what we eat. It may not always be on the food label, but there are five simple rules for identifying foods and cooking practices with a low AGE content:

> **Eat fresh and unprocessed foods.** Highly processed foods have much higher AGE levels when compared to their unprocessed counterparts, especially those processed foods that are crisped for flavour and texture (like biscuits, crisps, and crunchy cereals). These are baked at high temperature and high pressure, in which all water is quickly removed to get that extra crunch, which adds extra AGEs.

> **Water-based cooking.** Cooking in the presence of water or humidity (e.g. boiling, poaching, stewing, steaming, or using a slow cooker) is much better than frying, broiling, roasting or grilling. For example, a chicken breast fried in oil has five times the AGEs as the same chicken breast has when poached. Equally, an egg fried in butter contains four times the AGE levels as the same egg when it is boiled. One has only to look at the primarily water-based Asian cooking practices and the smooth face of an elderly Japanese person to understand this potential link.

> **Slow cooking.** Cooking on a low heat (less than 250°C) is better than at a higher temperature, which creates more AGEs over a shorter time than cooking at lower temperatures for longer periods of time.

> **Find flavour from sources other than the cooking process.** We all love flavour in our food. A low-AGE diet should not mean eating food devoid of flavour. It simply means we get flavour from sources other than browning (e.g. from herbs and spices) or choose products that have great natural flavours. We really don't need to fry, barbecue, roast or broil to get meat tasting great. In fact, marinating foods may reduce AGE formation while still creating incredible flavourful meals.

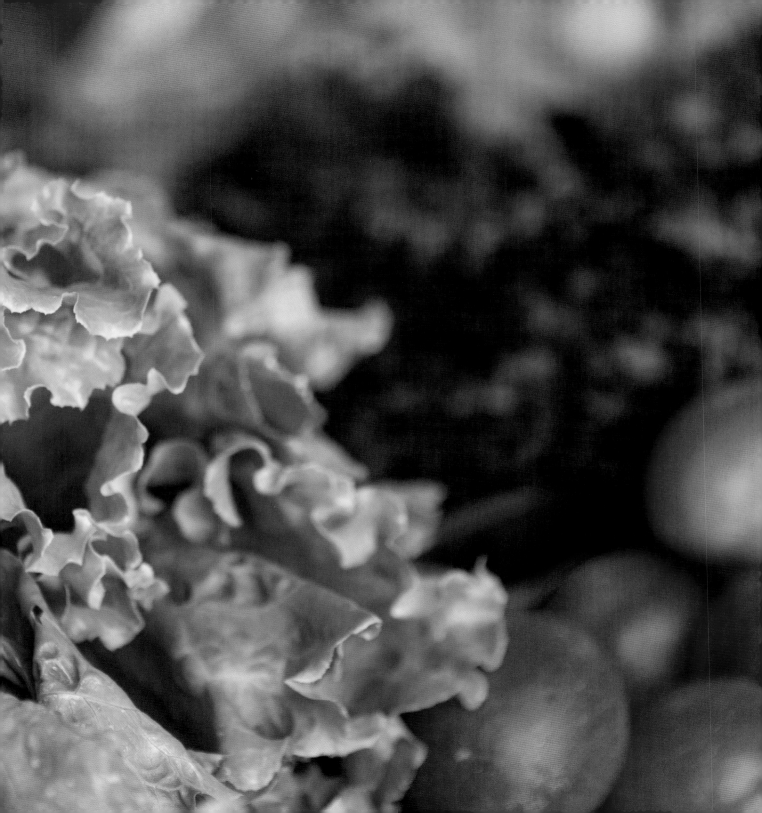

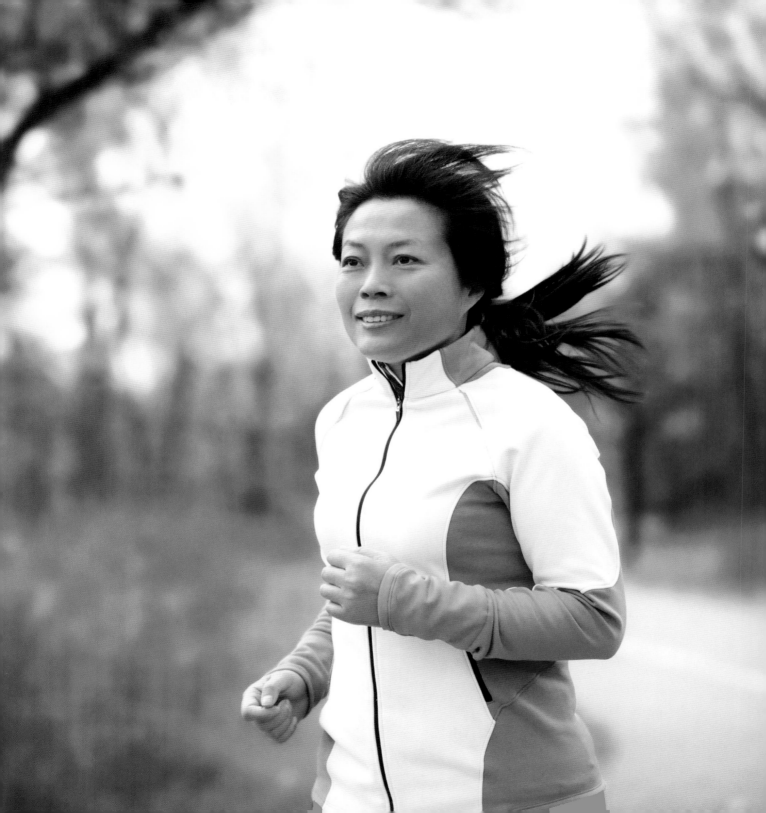

CHAPTER 12
EXERCISE AND SKIN

Regular physical activity is critical for our health, but many of us scarcely get any. The Western world is afflicted by a very sedentary lifestyle, whether at work or at home. Couch potatoes have an increased risk of diabetes, obesity, high blood pressure, heart disease, and some cancers compared to those who undertake regular physical activity. While it can seem difficult to get exercise when many of us spend our working hours sitting at a desk in front of a computer, remember that just 30 minutes of exercise a day can have extremely beneficial effects (or invest in a stand-up desk; it can really boost your health).

It is true, the fit survive. Their skin looks better too. In particular, resistance training has multiple benefits including the maintenance of muscle mass, stimulating the secretion of growth hormone and enhancing metabolic activity. Increasing our lean muscle mass can also improve skin tone. As we age, our skin loses its plumpness due in part to loss of muscle tone. So if we can build up lean muscle, we'll get a volumising effect in our skin.

MYOKINES

There is good evidence that physical exercise has a number of direct and indirect benefits on our skin. The obvious one is burning calories that would otherwise be deposited under our skin. Muscle activity also releases chemical signals, known as myokines, which promote skin health. Indeed, the lack of this regular chemical stimulus from muscles is one reason why skin ageing is accelerated in sedentary people. Vigorous exercise also makes us hot, which stimulates blood flow to the skin (creating the well-known flush of exercise). When repeated, the skin adapts by improving its blood flow to more efficiently cope with the future effects of exercise. This improvement in blood flow also benefits the health of our skin. Finally, regular physical activity improves many aspects of psychological health, including self-esteem and emotional well-being. If we feel great, we also look great.

TAKING IT 'SLOW'

It is beyond the scope of this chapter to detail how to become more physically active, and more importantly remain that way. There are no overnight solutions. The best way is to take it 'slow', by doing what's right for each of us, by getting help, by defining clear and achievable goals, by eliminating the negative and accenting the positive, and by focusing on the long term rather than a temporary quick fix.

FACIAL EXERCISES

Lines and creases don't happen just anywhere on our faces. They occur in very specific spots, primarily around the eyes and mouth and on the chin and forehead. These are areas of skin that have been stretched repeatedly, year after year, by the habitual movements of our faces. It is a bit of an old wives' tale that we shouldn't squint or make faces, in case this expression gets stuck on our face (when the wind changes). It may well be that years of mirth and laughter have given us laugh-lines or years of worry have given us frown lines. People who are grumpy and hostile throughout their lives are more likely to look mad even when they are not trying. Ultimately our faces reflect how we repeatedly use them.

When the muscles of the face contract, the skin creases at right angles to the direction of this movement, but when we are young it bounces back and looks smooth again. With repeated movement, and the loss of elasticity as we age, we slowly develop permanent changes in the skin that form horizontal lines, at first small but gradually larger and deeper.

We don't all smile the same way. Some people hardly smile at all while others beam from ear to ear. Our wrinkles are therefore as unique as the face that wears them. For most people, the lines on their face tell a story. The problem comes if these lines become fixed. We might not be feeling grumpy or tired, but our lines paint a different picture. Fixing this incongruity is one of the most common reasons why people use cosmetic procedures.

One common recommendation for the treatment of wrinkles is facial exercises. These are sometimes referred to as face yoga, face pilates, facial toning or facial aesthetics.

The exercises attempt to relax the muscles of our face by pulling faces that are 'larger than life', but there is really no evidence that it works to reduce wrinkles. They can improve blood flow to the face, which may be good for you (and can be achieved by massaging your face for just 10 minutes or so, which also helps you relax). People who do these facial exercises often report feeling younger, however, so it probably doesn't matter if it has a concrete physiological effect.

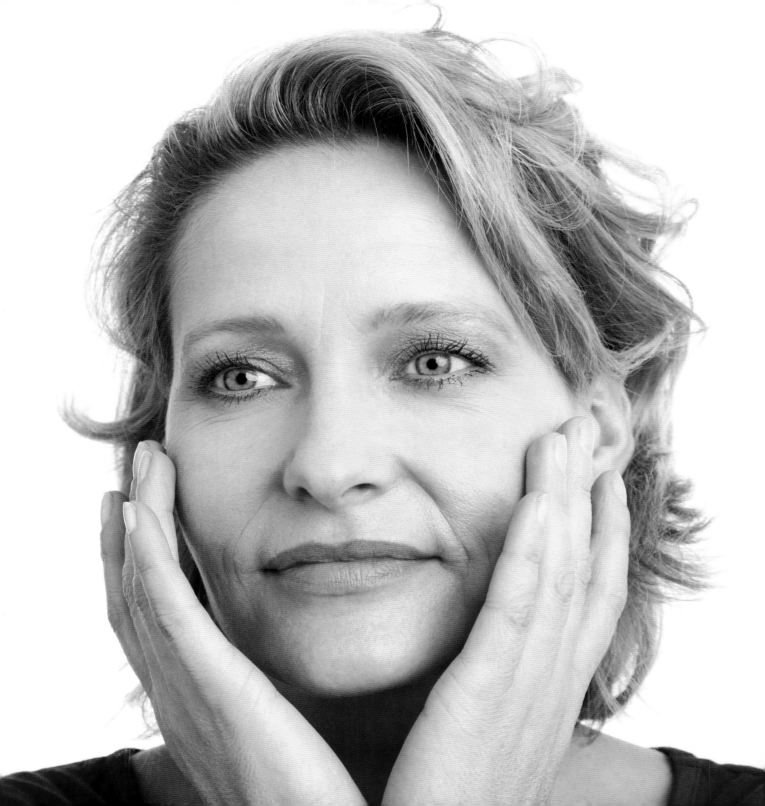

CHAPTER 13

SKIN MICROBIOME AND PREBIOTICS

Our skin plays host to an enormous and diverse microbial population. Each square centimetre of our skin is home to approximately 10 million bacteria. These bugs are not just hitchhiking along for the ride, but rather they pay their way by performing a number of mutually beneficial functions. Importantly, they prevent more damaging bacteria from getting a foothold. In fact, they actively fight them off, forming a key part of our skin's defence against infection. Some skin bacteria actually release chemicals that assist in moisturising the skin and protecting it against sunlight.

DYSBIOSIS

Imbalance of bacteria on our skin (known as dysbiosis) can occur when external or internal factors mean our happy residents get replaced by less hospitable bacteria. Dysbiosis plays a role in several skin diseases, including psoriasis, acne and dermatitis. There is also emerging evidence that the balance of bugs on our skin can contribute to how our skin ages. For example, low-level inflammation associated with sunlight, smoking and other environmental toxins may be enhanced by dysbiosis. Conversely, our healthy resident bacteria release chemicals to keep inflammation in check.

The chemical composition of oils that coat the outer surface of our skin (known as sebum) is also partly determined by the composition of bugs that grow in it and live off it. As discussed in chapter 3, sebum has a major role in determining the appearance of the skin. This is partly through its function of reducing water loss from the skin's surface. Too much sebum can lead to acne as pores become blocked, while too little sebum means the skin becomes dry and cracked and pores can get larger to compensate. It's a fine balance for which, in part, we have to thank our resident skin bacteria for maintaining.

The common fear of bacterial infection has led to a huge increase in antimicrobial cosmetic products – everything from soaps and rinses to makeup. However, at present there is no clear evidence that the ecology of the resident bacteria on our skin is changed significantly by the use of such products; however, the effects of their long-term use are still under investigation. For most of us, antibacterials on our skin are completely unnecessary. We would do much better using a moisturising soap.

Given the important role bacteria play in the skin, a number of studies have tried to induce a better balance in the skin's bacterial population by feeding them with beneficial chemicals. These chemicals are known as prebiotics, and have been successfully used for treating skin conditions like acne. Recent studies have also explored the effects of either eating beneficial bacteria or applying them directly to the skin. These are called probiotics, and are widely used in gastrointestinal health. Lactobacilli and bifidobacterium species of bacteria in yoghurt and other dairy products are well known, but their effect on the skin has only recently started to be investigated. However, some early studies have shown that changing our skin's bacteria balance can change our susceptibility to sun damage. In the future, our skin regimen may include taking anti-ageing bacteria every day, or applying chemicals to help the good guys do their job. That day is not yet here. In the meantime, we should probably not kill them off unnecessarily.

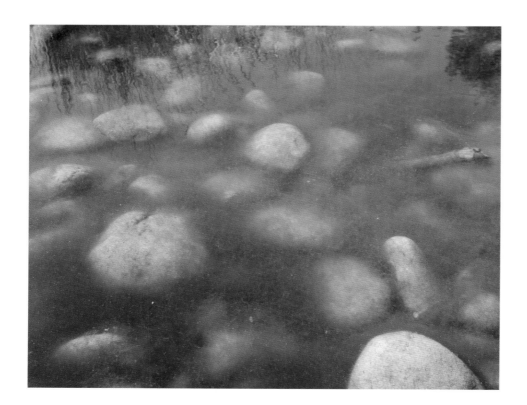

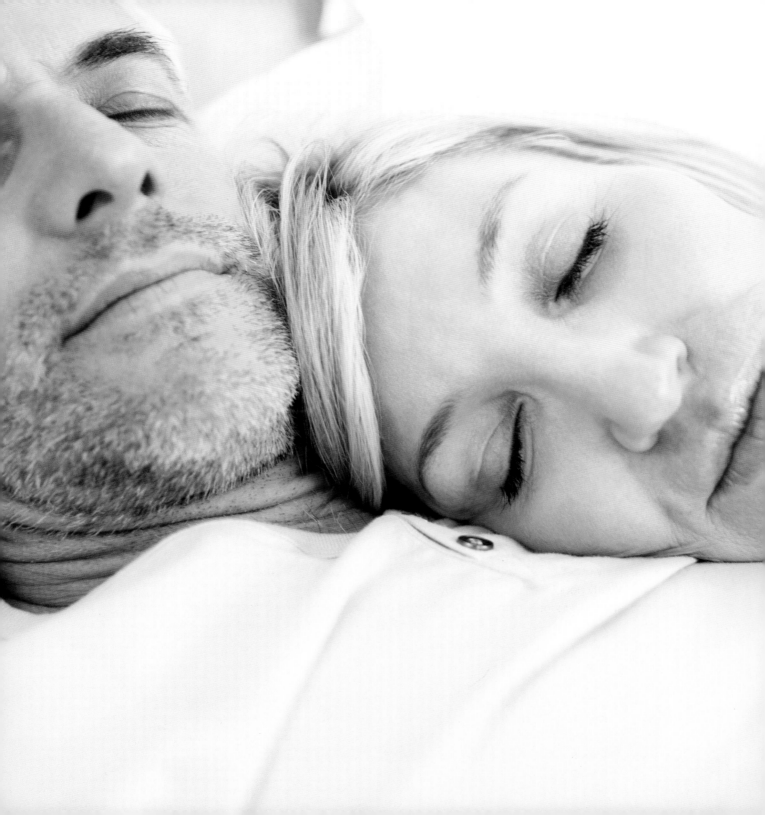

CHAPTER 14

SLEEP AND ITS IMPACT ON AGEING SKIN

It is often said that there is nothing like a good night's sleep for health and rejuvenation. After a night without rest, maybe with a young child at home or pulling an all-nighter, it's easy to understand why they call it 'beauty sleep'. Without a good night's sleep, we just don't look or feel that great in the morning. Neither does our skin. It looks tired and pale, lacking in lustre. Wrinkles, bags under the eyes and dark circles around them appear more pronounced. Studies show that even after only one night of missed sleep, others view our face as less attractive, less happy and less healthy. In other words, we look older. With chronic sleep deprivation, these changes become more marked and more persistent. Therefore, if we look after our sleep, we also look after our beauty.

Sleep is an important time for skin repair, when old and damaged cells and matrix are replaced with new organised matrix and younger, healthier cells. Blood flow to the skin increases during the night to support this function. Missing sleep and disrupting the biological rhythms associated with it will disrupt this process of rejuvenation. For example, wound healing and the skin's immune function are impaired when deprived of sleep but bolstered by a good night's rest.

Although it is widely suggested that an average of eight hours of sleep per night is best, there is no magic number that suits everyone. The amount of sleep needed varies between people, between seasons, and even over the course of the working week. As we get older, we tend to need less sleep on average, although healthy active elderly people will probably enjoy as much sleep as many younger adults. The simplest way to judge whether you are getting enough sleep is to see how you feel in the morning. If you wake up still tired, and are lethargic or find yourself dozing off through the day, you probably need to get more sleep.

SOLUTIONS FOR BETTER BEAUTY SLEEP

Just because sleep is an unconscious activity doesn't mean we have no control over it. There are many things we can do while we are awake to influence the quality and quantity our sleep. This is sometimes called 'sleep hygiene', but it is essentially eliminating those things that prevent natural sleep, while accentuating the positive triggers for sleep.

FACTORS THAT CAN INFLUENCE SLEEP

CONTEXT	RATIONALE
Darkness	Block out the light from the street or the next room and use bulbs that block blue light to maximise the melatonin surge that occurs with sleep. Keep the TV and computer out of the bedroom.
Coolness	Falling body temperature is an important cue for sleep. This can be enhanced by keeping our bedroom cooler than the rest of the house, or by having a bath or shower in the evening.
Quiet	Noise and stimulation are supposed to keep us awake. The bedroom should therefore be a quiet place.
Routine	When possible, we should try to go to bed, and wake up, at the same times each day, even on the weekends. This makes it easier to fall asleep at night and get up in the morning. Do the same things each time, like taking a shower, and include some 'mental cleaning' and relaxation into your daily sleep routine.
Comfort	Our bed should be a comfortable place. We spend more of our lifetime there than any other single place, but beds seldom receive as much attention as our car or the television. Simple things can help, such as regularly replacing worn out, uneven or uncomfortable mattress and pillows with those that allow us to maintain an anatomically neutral position.
No stimulation	For sleep to occur, we need to wind down so that our brains can enter the sleep cycle. Our brains cannot do this if they are trying to do something else, whether coping with stress or engaging in mental or physical activity. Taking caffeine (in coffee, tea, chocolate, cola or energy drinks) any time after 2 p.m. can see the buzz staying round until bedtime. Similarly, late meals can keep the brain going. Exercising within three hours of bedtime is also not recommended, as exercise releases hormones that keep us awake. Where possible, put work away at least an hour or two before bed. Use the bed only for sleeping, sex and relaxing activities such as reading.
Sunshine	Often, we see people out walking or running in the mornings – and far from indicating insomnia, morning exercise is actually one of the best ways to promote sound sleep. Not only is it a great way to reinforce our body clocks, but physical activity also works to enhance deep sleep. Morning sun is also lower in UVB, so it is safer for our skin.
Sex	Sexual activity can exert powerful positive influences over sleep patterns (although stressing over it won't help).

CONTEXT	RATIONALE
Stress management	One of the most important influences on our modern sleep patterns is stress. This can be emotional, physical or environmental stress, but the result is almost always a bad night's sleep. When stress is the culprit, the cause, not the symptoms, must be treated.
Enjoyment	Sleep is not the enforced laying down of tools. We can get so caught up in our work and our world (to finish that last page, or movie) that going to bed while still engaged is a punishment for adults as much as it is for our kids. With appropriate scheduling and spacing of our days, a sleep routine can be very enjoyable (whether it involves sex, a bedtime story, or a clean set of sheets) as well as very healthy.
Waking must be positive	There is nothing more irritating than a loud alarm clock that scares us awake. This rude awakening can damage our memories and learning, focus and attention, as well as our mood. An established sleep pattern always includes a healthy waking pattern.
Food and drink	Some foods can help us with a better night's sleep, including tryptophan-rich foods, including dairy (remember the glass of warm milk before bed) nuts and seeds, honey and eggs. However, caffeine, chocolate, and alcohol can delay sleep or reduce its quality.

WHAT ARE SLEEP LINES?

The downside of sleep may be wrinkles caused by sleeping on our front or side with our face buried in the pillow. Even though we usually roll around throughout the night, it's normal to spend much of the time asleep in the same, favourite position. Given the amount of time we spend asleep in bed, some practitioners believe that the position we favour to sleep in can influence how we look in the morning. Over many years this position can cause creases to form in the face and neck where the skin is bunched up in contact with a pillow. Some women report that sleeping on one particular side may even have put wrinkles in one of their breasts.

The obvious way to prevent such lines is to sleep on our back, but this is uncomfortable for many women, especially those with back problems or those who are prone to snoring. Some nifty pillows are available that not only help us sleep, but also keep us cool. Some pillows claim to prevent wrinkles, while supposedly wrinkle-busting sleep masks are also available and claim to act by cushioning the sleep-squashed skin. Whether these actually work is unclear, but certainly a decent pillow will help. Also many cosmetic practitioners recommend a satin or silk pillowcase to reduce friction on facial skin during sleep.

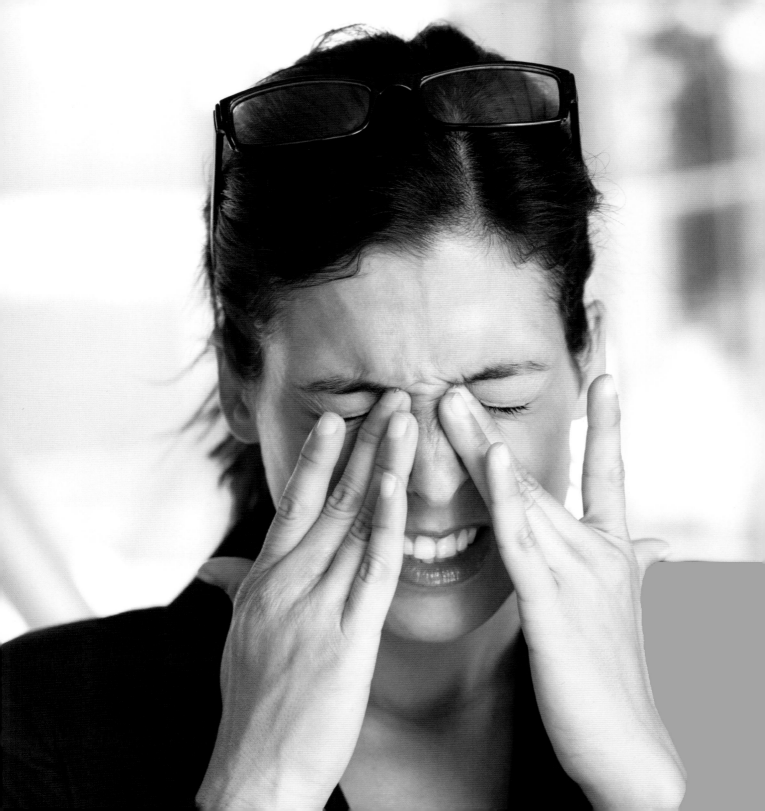

CHAPTER 15

STRESS PROMOTES SKIN AGEING

Everyday lives are filled with many challenges, and it is often said that we wear our stress on our faces. We call them 'worry lines' for a good reason. It's not just that these wrinkles accentuate the expression that we have when we are worried; stress really can leave a permanent mark on our face. Our skin is, in this sense, the mirror of our soul.

Stress triggers a range of responses in the body to defend against, cope with and adapt to it. These include the production of stress hormones, inflammatory cytokines, increased levels of cortisol (which hampers the immunity function of the skin) and activation of the sympathetic nervous system. The intensity of our response is determined not only by the intensity of the stress, but also by a host of other factors including context, genes, gender, previous experiences, coping skills and personality traits, as well as age itself.

These stress response pathways can also have major effects on the skin, such as reducing barrier functions, moisture content and matrix synthesis, and increasing inflammation in the skin. It is well known, for example, that skin problems like acne, psoriasis and eczema can often flare up when people with these conditions are stressed.

There is also data implicating stress in the process of ageing itself. For example, exposure to chronic stress is associated with shorter telomeres, the little bits on the end of chromosomes that indicate how old a cell is (and how long it has got to go). People who are exposed to stress don't just look older; they actually are older.

MANAGING STRESS

Life is full of stress. Don't ignore it. As part of our plan to look after our skin as we get older, we should take time to recognise causes of stress and find ways to manage it better. There are many different ways to handle stress, too many to discuss in detail in this chapter. Each will be suited to particular situations and particular people. Some people will need more help than others, based on their resilience and the weight of their burden. Chances are, however, we will all need to work on our stress levels, sooner or later.

Some things we can do ourselves, others we undertake with the help of various health practitioners. Some of the most effective stress management techniques include formal psychotherapy, time management training, relaxation training, meditation, mind-body techniques, mindful breathing, biofeedback, hypnosis, yoga, tai chi, exercise, mindfulness meditation, guided imagery and taking time out. Gardening or music can be equally effective in reducing stress. When used routinely each can serve to build resilience to stress, but it's not the same for everyone. Not everyone can do yoga. Not everyone likes gardening or music. There is no simple answer. The most effective strategies are the ones we enjoy, the ones that put our mind at ease, the ones we can fit into our schedule and the ones we want to do again and again.

Identifying the sources of stress in our life is an important step. Be aware of your environment and your life inside its bubble. For example, time management skills come from identifying the burdens of our workload and creating a balanced, effective approach to either meeting that workload or changing it. Equally, conflict resolution comes from recognising both the impasse and finding a mutually satisfactory way to solve the conflict. In other cases, disclosure of stress (such as abuse) can be an important initial step in its management.

Another key component is to identify those factors that are central to controlling our stress. From self-awareness comes self-control and other forms of mental discipline required to cope with stress. Just reflecting on what is good in our life can help, because we know where to go to find things that make us feel happy and energised.

While some resolve can be found within, external support is also important. People who age well (and are less stressed) tend to stay connected with the world. It may be that a lack of stress allows this to occur, or that robust support allows some people to better cope with stress. One way to improve our outlook is to cultivate a support network. Join a club. Find a partner. Stay close to children and friends.

Changing the way stress is perceived can also modify its impact. If we think we are stressed, then we are. When we recognise that we have the resources to cope, stress is no longer such a threat. Some of this 'stress resilience' comes down to confidence, the learning of coping skills, or developing a positive outlook. These can be cultivated and fostered over time and with practice. The stress-resilient person may have the same stress factors as other people (e.g. the traffic) but they will expect everything will be okay in the end, and is in a better position to deal with stress simply because they know that they have the tools to deal with it. A number of studies have shown that simply learning to 'accentuate the positive' is associated with reduced stress. Optimism can be learned with practice and become an integral part of our life.

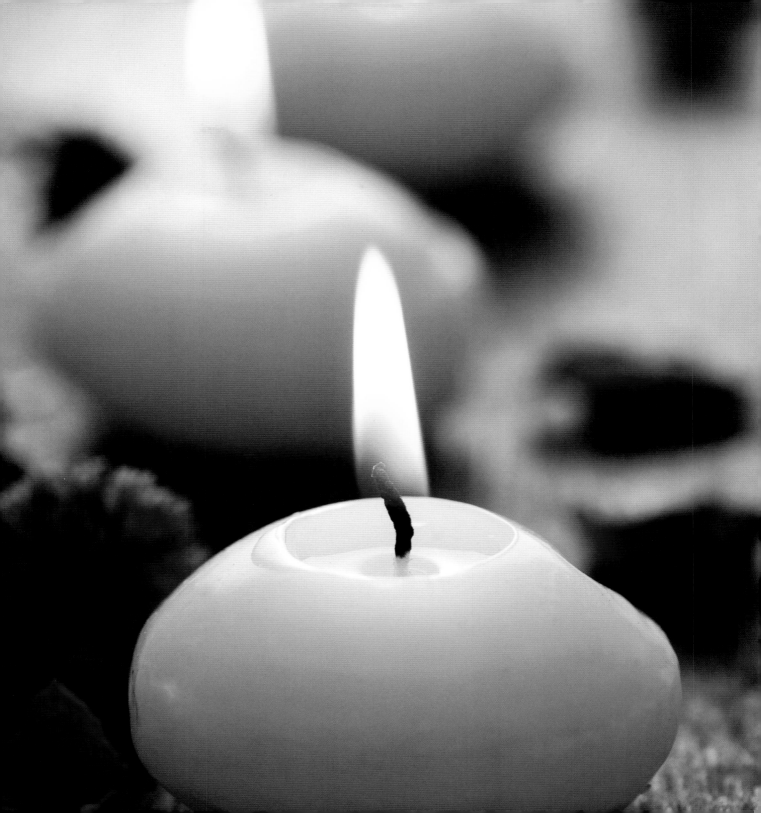

SECTION 5

HORMONES

CHAPTER 16: HORMONES AND THEIR IMPACT ON THE AGEING PROCESS

Ageing well is all about achieving and maintaining balance. The job of balancing the chemical processes of the body (known as metabolism) is performed by hormones.

As we age there is a substantial decline in these functions, due to decreased levels of hormones or their inadequate regulation. It also results in significant changes in our skin. There are many and varied hormones that impact the skin including the sex hormones, growth hormone and melatonin, our sleep hormone.

Menopause is when we often start to notice accelerated changes in hormones. As we get closer to menopause, we typically get an increase in facial hair, while our skin sags, may get oilier or drier, and its elasticity declines. The epidermis can become thinner and we become more prone to sun damage, hyperpigmentation and age spots. Hormone modulation can help enormously and is well worth looking at if you want to be strategic in managing these changes.

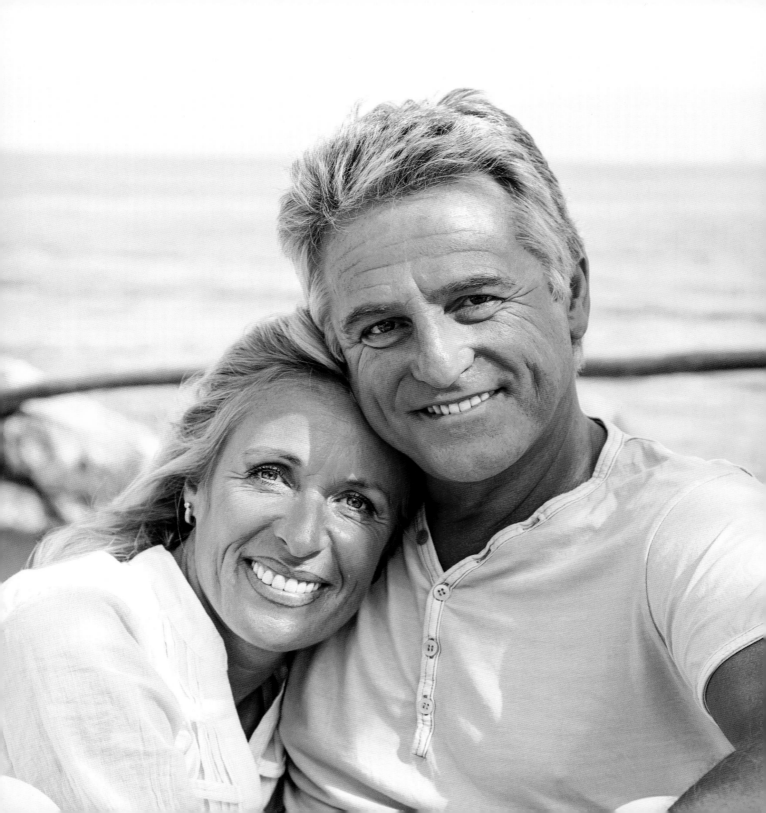

HORMONES AND THEIR IMPACT ON THE AGEING PROCESS

Ageing can wreak havoc on our hormones. Some hormones decrease while others increase with age. Hormones need to be balanced in order for our bodies to function optimally and particularly for women in their mid- to late-forties, a natural transition occurs in the way the sex hormones like oestrogen and progesterone are produced and released, which can knock this balance off kilter.

MENOPAUSE

Over the course of five to ten years before menopause (known as peri-menopause), hormone production slows, becomes more erratic and eventually shuts down altogether. This is due to the exhaustion of oestrogen-producing reserves in the ovaries. During the latter part of this transition, cycle lengths become irregular and menstruation eventually stops, which is what is referred to as the menopause.

The effects of the ovaries shutting down does not just impact upon reproductive functioning; it changes almost every aspect of a woman's body, including the skin, which can become more prone to thinning, dryness and roughness, bruising, wrinkling and slow healing.

For women who suffer menopausal symptoms, hormone replacement therapy (HRT) can be highly effective. In addition, there is now data showing that HRT can result in improvement in the skin. HRT is available in a number of different forms, which can be delivered by oral, transdermal (cream, troches) or vaginal means. Women who have not had a hysterectomy are usually given a 'combined' regimen, in which oestrogen is delivered alongside progestogen, to avoid the development of endometrial cancer. This combination can be taken on a cyclical basis (like the contraceptive pill) or on a continuous daily schedule.

TOPICAL OESTROGENS

Some women have looked to topical oestrogens in cosmeceuticals as a way to both balance hormones and preserve the skin's appearance. Only oestriol should be used topically as it targets dermal receptors. This can modestly impact upon the skin's appearance – including a reduction in wrinkle depth – mostly by stimulating matrix regrowth and increasing the skin's water content. Importantly, topical oestriol will not affect blood levels, so the risks of cancer and heart disease are minimal.

A number of so-called 'natural alternatives' to oestrogen are also used in cosmeceuticals. For example, plants like soy, clover, flax and hops contain chemicals that are able to bind and partially activate oestrogen receptors. These are called phytoestrogens. The most popular phyto-oestrogen additives to skincare products include genistein and other soy isoflavones. Although many have antioxidant effects, in general these are less effective and less potent than naturally occurring human oestrogens.

TESTOSTERONE

Blood levels of the major male hormones (called androgens) decline by about one percent each year from our mid-thirties onwards. This is called the 'andropause' and occurs in both men and women. Women in their forties have on average half the testosterone level they had in their twenties. Sometimes, androgen levels may be low enough to reduce quality of life, resulting in symptoms including reduced libido, fatigue, disturbed sleep, concentration and mood, pelvic-floor problems and 'middle-age spread.' It can also affect the health of the skin, contributing to wrinkling and reduced elasticity.

Supplementation with testosterone may be an option for women, but there can be side effects. These include acne, increased facial hair and weight gain, breast enlargement and changes in mood (including increased levels of aggression when taken in high doses). When used in appropriate doses, testosterone does not cause women to look and behave like men (though transgender women have used high doses of the hormone to aid transition).

DHEA

The body also has a buffer to make sure that it can keep making sex hormones. These are pro-hormones like dehydroepiandrosterone (DHEA) and its sulphated derivative (DHEAS), which can be converted as required into either testosterone or oestrogen. In common with other hormones, DHEA levels decline as we age, and can result in fatigue, loss of libido and decline in skin quality. It is also associated with an increased risk of heart disease, depression and cognitive impairment.

If you have low levels of DHEA, taking supplements can significantly improve quality of life. However, there are potential side effects, such as oilier-than-normal hair and skin, acne, hair loss and increased facial hair due to extra testosterone production.

GROWTH HORMONE

Growth hormone is a key regulator in the human body, acting to build up and maintain structures in all parts of the body, including the skin. As we age, growth slows and eventually stops. Levels of growth hormone decline every year from puberty onwards. This is known as the somatopause. By the time we reach 70 years of age, growth hormone levels are about one-fifth of what they were at the age of 30.

Of all the hormonal changes that occur in the human body, the decline in growth hormone levels is the most closely correlated with ageing. In fact, some people who have a reduced capability to make growth hormone (through genetics, disease or injury) typically manifest many of the signs and symptoms of premature ageing, including heart disease, bone thinning, expanding waistlines, cognitive decline and characteristic skin changes.

MELATONIN

Melatonin is a natural hormone, released according to the body's natural rhythms, with the highest levels occurring at night and the lowest levels around the middle of the day. This cycling of melatonin is important for the regulation of sleep and for aligning other parts of our circadian rhythms. Melatonin also has a number of important, independent effects on health and ageing, including effects on oxidative stress, the immune system and inflammation. It also influences the functions of the skin, such as augmenting hair growth and reducing sun damage. Unfortunately, the production of melatonin declines with age. In fact, some elderly people show little or no nocturnal increase in melatonin production. This can make getting to sleep a problem, and it is also likely to have an impact on skin.

SECTION 6:
SKINCARE

Skincare products that contain 'active ingredients' are called cosmeceuticals. They have both cosmetic and pharmaceutical properties. A cosmeceutical is a topical agent that does more than makeup, with effects on appearance that last longer. It also means something less than a bone fide pharmaceutical treatment or cosmetic procedure, which are regulated to meet strict medical standards for evidence and use.

There is now unequivocal scientific evidence that the regular application of cosmeceuticals, including retinoids, antioxidants, emollients, peptides, vitamins, hormones, phytochemicals and many other active agents, improve skin's appearance and/or prevent its deterioration.

Cosmeceuticals is one of the fastest growing sections of the skincare market, especially the anti-ageing industry. It seems that on an almost weekly basis a new exotic combination of ingredients claims to produce ageless skin. The catch is that no scientific proof is required for cosmeceuticals to be sold as cosmetics. Indeed, any claims of effectiveness would necessitate costly testing and regulation, requiring sales only on prescription or by a pharmacy.

This contributes to the confusing labelling in cosmeceuticals; what they can say they do versus what they might actually do for our skin. In fact, some skin treatments are available both as prescription and over-the-counter cosmetic products (the latter usually in very low concentrations or potency formulations), blurring the distinction between cosmeceuticals and pharmaceuticals further.

In addition, it is commonly assumed that because a cosmetic contains an ingredient, that ingredient will penetrate the skin and have an effect. Otherwise, why use it? However, the prime function of the skin is to act as a barrier, keeping anything in the external environment out. Professor Johann Wiechers, Professor of Pharmacy and consultant to many large cosmetic companies, estimates that less than one percent of active ingredients in cosmetics enter the skin. This is because most cosmetic companies don't test for active ingredients entering the skin or even if cosmetic products have any objective effects.

Some companies use ingredient supplier's results, which can be misleading. Results can be cherry picked, may have differing formulations or be unreliable. The best way to be sure of a product's effectiveness is to look for those with medically proven data to back up their claims. Don't just rely on the ingredients list for your information.

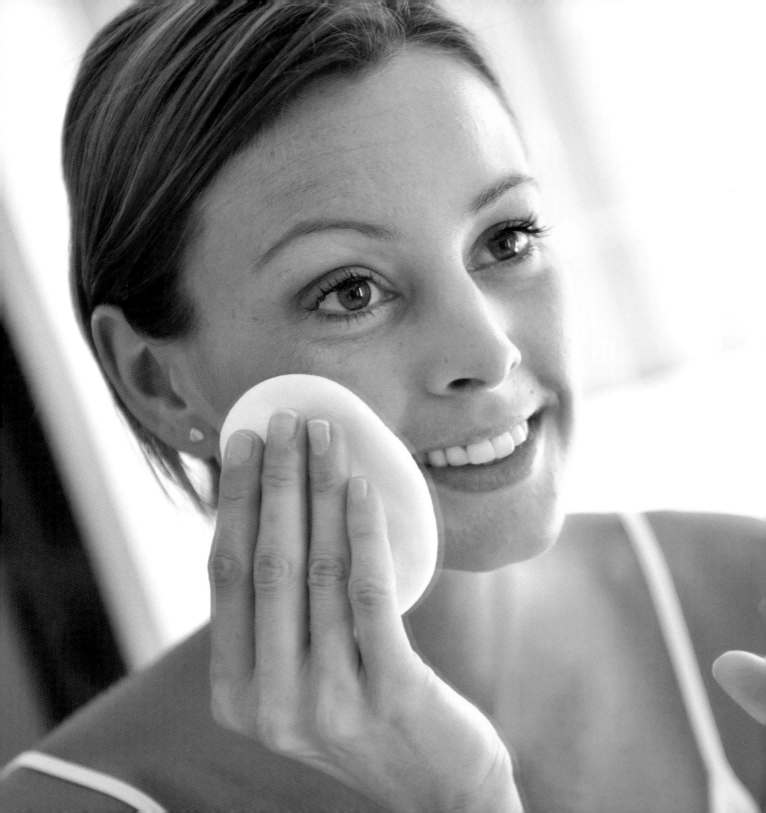

Cleansing and exfoliating are the mainstays of a good skin regimen, with toning being an optional step for many women.

CLEANSERS

Regular use of skin cleansers should be an integral part of every woman's skincare regimen. Cleansers remove grime, makeup and oil, and so improve the appearance of our skin. Regular cleansing also has the potential to improve the health of our skin. However, the injudicious use of cleansers can actually strip beneficial elements from our skin and promote skin damage, inflammation and ageing. In particular, strong soaps and detergents remove the natural oils that form an important part of the skin's barrier function. Less oil means the skin's ability to hold water will be reduced, making it appear less full and more prone to wrinkles.

The regular use of cleansers really came into modern cosmetic practice in response to the failure of soap to meet our skincare needs. Traditionally, soap was highly alkaline and very irritating to our skin. It also didn't smell good. It left the skin irritated, dried, and prone to wrinkles and lines. Using cleansing products became the only solution, and many cosmetic companies were founded on that premise.

This same argument does not hold today. Some modern soaps and soap substitutes really do provide effective and gentle cleansing. The problem is, in a vast sea of products, to find one suitable for your needs. The alternative that the cosmetic industry offers is to use a specific skin-sensitive cleansing agent.

Broadly speaking, cleansing agents are water-based, alcohol-based or oil-based. Oil- and alcohol-based cleansers are more suited to oily skins where they do an excellent job of removing excess oil and any makeup, dirt and grime trapped in it. Whether or not we use a mild soap or a commercial-grade cleanser, every time we cleanse, to a greater or lesser extent we lose some natural oils. This is why the use of an emollient (occlusive) moisturiser (chapter 18) every time after cleansing is recommended.

EXFOLIATION

Skin cleansing sometimes deliberately involves removing the rough layer of dead skin cells that forms the outermost layer of the skin. These cells will fall off of their own accord eventually, but as we age this process slows down. Some treatments can help these dead skin cells detach and fall off. These are known as exfoliation, resurfacing, peeling or refreshing.

Removing the old, dead cells on the surface achieves a 'lustre' or 'gloss' effect on our skin, as the underlying cells revealed after exfoliation are moisture rich, more reflective and more uniform. Removing the outer layer of dead cells that covers our skin also accelerates the process of exfoliation. In other words, if we lose skin on the outside, our skin responds by making more skin cells deep inside to compensate for the loss. This drives younger, plumper cells to the surface and their greater moisture content makes the skin look and feel younger.

Many of the active ingredients that are used in chemical peels (which act as exfoliants) are also used in many facial cleansers, moisturisers and toners, albeit in tiny concentrations, about a hundred-fold lower than in chemical peels. This means we can safely use them to gently exfoliate our skin on a daily basis.

Exfoliants were probably the first facial cosmeceuticals and have been used by women for skin rejuvenation for thousands of years. Cleopatra's preferred combination of sour milk, grape peel and lemon juice has been replaced in modern times by the actual active ingredients contained in each of them – alpha-hydroxy acids (AHAs), tartaric acid and citric acid, respectively. To these traditional ingredients we have added new AHAs, such as glycolic acid. Even though many AHAs are found naturally in nature, today almost all AHAs in cosmetic products are made in a laboratory. All AHAs work in the same way to remove excess dead cells from the skin's surface, stimulate healing and turnover, and allow new skin cells to emerge by replacing the old and damaged skin, thus improving skin texture, colour and appearance.

The trick is to find out which formulation has the best effects on your skin with the least irritation. It's mostly trial and error, although experienced practitioners will usually have a good idea what will work on your skin.

When the outer layer of the skin is shed, this can lead to increased sensitivity to sunlight. It is often suggested that exfoliants should be used in the evening, so the skin can regenerate through the night. Remember that using exfoliants means we should be especially vigilant with sun protection.

Instead of chemicals or soaps, some anti-ageing skincare regimens utilise good old-fashioned scrubbing, using textured cloths or creams than contain particles such as microbeads. This is more or less the same principle used in dermabrasion (see chapter 26) – to mechanically detach old, dead cells from the surface of the skin to let the younger, healthier ones come through. Scrubbing is often combined with the application of low concentrations of exfoliants to make the process even more effective. It is recommended that you scrub perpendicular to the direction of your wrinkles, as you don't want to make the ruts deeper.

Scrubbing does have its downsides, however. Many abrasive implements such as loofahs, pumice stones and sea sponges can harbour nasty bugs. Some scrubs can also actually scratch holes in the skin and this can lead to acne, sensitive skin, or broken blood vessels. Microbeads also have a major environmental impact that should not be ignored, adding to oceanic and terrestrial pollution levels.

A number of modern cosmetic cleansers contain enzymes that have the potential to promote exfoliation by digesting the protein bonds that hold skin cells together. These enzymes are usually derived from exotic plants like papaya, pineapple or pomegranate. They are often advertised as being less irritable than AHAs, especially for women with sensitive skin.

TONING

After cleansing (and before moisturising) it is often recommended to use a toner (or tonic). Toners are basically another form of cleanser, taking away the last of the makeup, dirt, bacteria and debris from the skin as well as any residual cleanser. Like cleanser, some toners also contain low concentrations of exfoliants to assist with the removal of dead skin cells and to restore pH balance after the use of a less-than-ideal alkaline soap.

Unfortunately, toners also remove some of the skin's natural oils and healthy bacteria. After vigorous cleansing, further toning can be very drying and reduce the skin's barrier function, even if immediately followed by a moisturiser. This is probably why most ageing women skip this step. Some toners actually contain moisturisers such as propylene glycol glycerine or sorbitol to deliberately counter this problem and allow for more broad use across a range of skin types.

Toners are usually alcohol-based. Putting concentrated alcohol on our skin's surface acts to cool the skin as the alcohol evaporates. This causes blood to divert away from the skin, temporarily creating a more even appearance, as differential blood flow is one of things that creates blotchiness in the skin. This cooling effect is also handy when considering the vigorous scrubbing of a cleansing regime can leave the skin hot, blotchy and itchy. Cooling the skin also gives the pleasing sensation of skin tightening, albeit only temporarily and without significant physical changes in the skin.

ASTRINGENTS

Some toners also contain chemicals that trigger the skin to shrink or contract. These are known as astringents. The most common ones are tannins from chamomile, witch-hazel (hamamelis), green tea and other herbs. Minerals like zinc, aluminium and copper also have astringent properties. Aromatic elements such as menthol, sage or camphor can stimulate the cold-sensing nerves in the skin, which causes surface blood vessels to constrict as if it were cold outside.

A common reason for recommending the use of an astringent is that it can temporarily reduce the size of your pores. This makes them less visible, and your skin tone more smooth and even. It is true that pores become more visible as we age and that the tightening of the skin after astringents makes pores less visible, but this is only a temporary effect and disappears rapidly when the toner evaporates. It is also often claimed that closing pores using astringents could stop subsequent makeup or moisturiser becoming stuck in pores, clogging them and leading to blackheads and other blemishes.

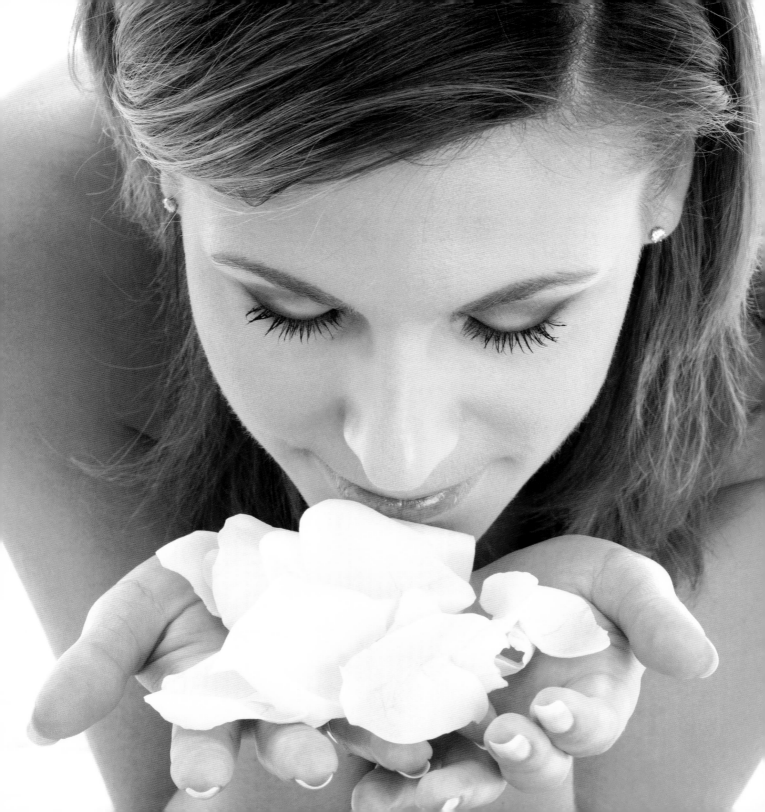

CHAPTER 18

MOISTURISING

Dry skin looks awful. It feels awful too. When the amount of water in our skin is reduced, lines and wrinkles become much more prominent. The skin's surface looks rough, dull and scaly, and we appear older as a result. The converse is also true. Old skin is often dry. This is because its moisture-holding properties are reduced and slower turnover of cells sees a build-up of bone-dry dead cells on the skin's surface. This is one of the reasons why daily efforts to increase or at the very least maintain water content in the skin through the regular use of moisturisers are an important part of any anti-ageing skincare strategy.

Increasing the water content of our skin makes it look fuller, softer, more luminous and younger. This is not just good for aesthetic reasons it is also important for our skin's health, as some areas of our skin become so dry that they can become inflamed, red, cracked, and itchy.

WHAT ARE MOISTURISERS AND HOW DO THEY WORK?

There are an enormous number of different products that are labelled as moisturisers. They include creams, ointments, soap substitutes and bath oils. Most of these are little more than a vehicle for delivering a fragrance and don't have much direct effect on our skin's health, especially in the dermis where we really need the help.

The right moisturisers, though, can make a real difference to how our skin looks and feels. This makes choosing the best moisturiser one of the most important decisions we will make for our skin's appearance. Most effective moisturisers work to increase the water content of our skin in one of three different ways:

> Occlusives or semi-occlusive moisturisers. These form a thin film on your skin to create a barrier that reduces the loss of moisture due to evaporation. The best-known examples include petrolatum, lanolin, mineral oil, soybean oil, grapeseed oil, and silicones like dimethicone. The downside is that the most effective occlusive moisturisers also feel the greasiest on our skin.

> Humectant moisturising creams. These contain chemicals that attract water into the drier outer layer of the skin and increase its water-holding capacity. As the outer layer of the skin swells, it makes the skin look smoother with fewer wrinkles and fine lines. Among the best-known examples include glycerine,

gelatine, panthenol, PCA, honey, sorbital and urea. Hyaluronic acid is the most potent humectant and forms a film on the skin. Humectants attract water directly from the atmosphere (if the humidity is greater than 80 percent). These products also pull water from deep within the skin out to the surface, and when moisture is nearer the surface, the risk of losing it by evaporation increases. This is why humectants are always combined with occlusives to enhance the water-holding capacity of the skin. The water-holding capacity of humectants is also critical to prevent cosmetic products from drying out on the shelf.

> **Emollients or barrier-repair agents.** These replace lipids (like cholesterol and ceramide), amino acids and/or oils in the sebum that normally act as a barrier to retain skin moisture, as well as contribute to the skin's natural flexibility and smoothness. They do this by filling the gaps and cracks between cells to create a smooth surface, and they also help to heal a damaged skin barrier. Emollients can also improve the stability of other active ingredients. Compared with occlusives that sit on the surface of the skin and provide only transient improvement, emollients can penetrate deeper to reach live skin cells, where they are incorporated into the skin.

Almost all commercial moisturisers contain a combination of occlusives, humectants and emollients, each in their own proprietary forms. Some moisturisers, like lanolin, function as an emollient, humectant and occlusive moisturiser at the same time.

THE BEST TIME TO USE MOISTURISERS

Rather than waiting for our skin to get dry, it pays to be proactive with moisturisers. Probably the best time to put on moisturisers is straight after a shower or bath, especially after you have used a skin cleanser that may temporarily reduce barrier function. Moisturisers should ideally be applied to slightly damp skin, which is then gently patted with a towel rather than rubbed dry.

In spa treatments (also called balneotherapy) that use hot baths, steam, mud or sand to cleanse the skin, oil is added to the water, and it coats your skin on the way out, sealing the moisture in. Alternatively, emollients are put on the skin immediately after leaving the bath. This means our wet skin stays wet, meaning it looks and feels plumper and more youthful.

SELECTING THE BEST MOISTURISER

All skin types can benefit from moisturisers, but the right type of moisturiser needs to be applied for your type. There are many reasons why a product may not work for you. These include an overly greasy feel, the smell, the stickiness, the shine, their unattractive look and the absorption rate. What we usually want is one that is not too greasy, and which spreads smoothly and easily.

The most expensive moisturisers are not necessarily the best. There are some really well-crafted moisturisers that contain old-fashioned ingredients that outperform many of the newfangled super-products. Just because it contains a particular active ingredient doesn't mean it will work the same when used in combination with other products in a skincare regimen.

Some skin can become irritated by certain chemical components. Sensitive skin should be spared fragrances, preservatives, dyes or acids. Another common problem can be flare-ups of acne, especially with predominantly occlusive preparations, which tend to block pores.

Moisturisers are often also a vehicle for delivering active components such as sunscreen (SPF), antioxidants, cosmeceuticals, botanicals, cell-communicators and other restorative agents.

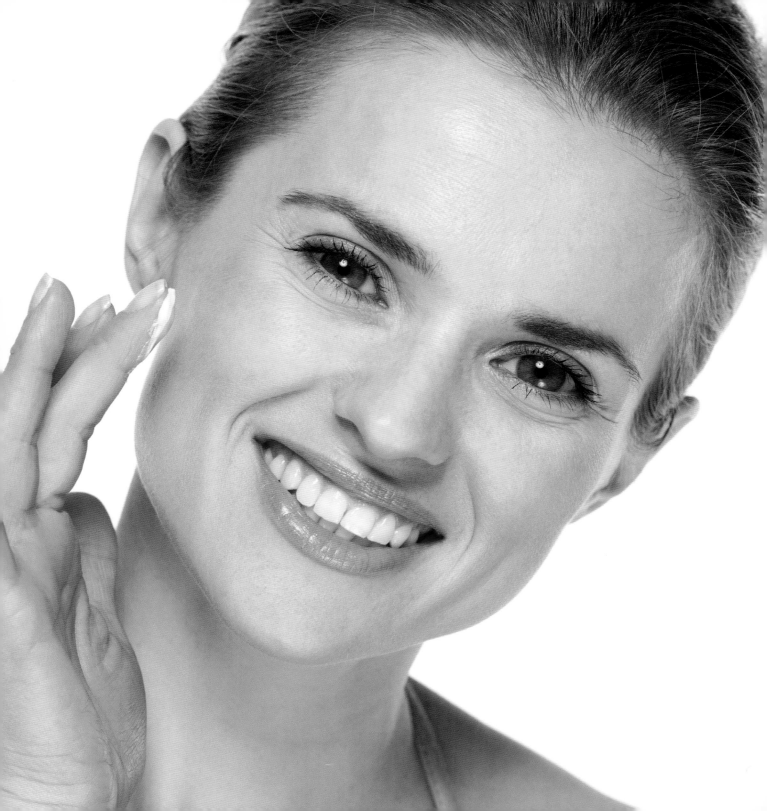

CHAPTER 19
TOPICAL ANTIOXIDANTS

Damage to our skin is partly driven by the generation of highly reactive and toxic free radicals. Damage caused by free radicals is a key trigger for inflammation and matrix breakdown in our skin, and hence wrinkles. Consequently, almost every cosmeceutical product now claims to contain some form of antioxidant (i.e. has the ability to destroy free radicals). Antioxidants do not, however, undo damage caused by free radicals. Free radicals react so fast and are so transitory that any antioxidant has to be right there at the moment of free radical generation to have any significant effect. For example, we often put on antioxidant creams after sun exposure. This will not reverse sun damage, although it will boost our natural protections against further damage.

There are many ways to fight off free radicals, including vitamins, minerals and hormones, and cosmeceuticals will usually include one or more types.

All antioxidants can neutralise free radicals in a test tube and as such, can be labelled as such on cosmetic products. Some do this better than others, which gives them kudos on the oxygen radical absorbance capacity (ORAC) scale. In theory, putting these antioxidants onto the skin so that they are there at the very moment that free radicals are generated, whether by sunlight, smoke, pollution or our metabolism, could reduce the chances of free radicals damaging our skin and contributing to ageing.

In practice, even though the label says 'contains antioxidants' it does not guarantee that the antioxidant qualities of this particular product – in combination with those fellow ingredients – have actually been tested. Most brands contain only very low concentrations of antioxidants. Getting antioxidants across the skin's barrier and into the places in the skin where the free radicals are actually being generated is also problematic with such products.

This said, there is some evidence that putting significant amounts of potent antioxidants on our skin can prevent the damage the results from oxidative stress, such as that caused by excessive sunlight or smoking. New delivery techniques and combinations may also partly offset the obvious limitations in skin penetration.

It is not known which antioxidant or combination is the most effective. Ascorbic acid and vitamin E combined have been shown to reduce the death (apoptosis) of epidermal cells when used with a sunscreen, compared to the same sunscreen used on its own. Look for evidence that a product reduces the effects of UV damage (by reducing the amount of damaged DNA) on the kind of skin we have (and not just on the hide of a research mouse!). However, as a general rule it is a good idea to look for products that contain a number of different antioxidants, to maximise the potential benefits. While there are thousands of different antioxidants, let's take a look at some of the more common ones, all of which can have similar benefits for skin rejuvenation.

POPULAR ANTIOXIDANTS

VITAMIN C (ASCORBATE, L-ASCORBIC ACID)

Vitamin C is naturally found in high levels in human skin, where it is taken up from the circulation and assists with maintaining a healthy epidermis. Vitamin C acts both as an antioxidant and a facilitator of matrix synthesis and stability. It is depleted in the skin following exposure to oxidising forces like sunlight and smoking. Ageing also sees a decline in our skin's vitamin C levels. Vitamin C-rich products, when in the right formulation, can help to reverse some of the results of ageing.

There is only one true form of vitamin C and many derivatives, some of which absorb into the skin better than others. The derivatives include magnesium ascorbyl phosphate, sodium ascorbyl phosphate and ascorbyl tetraisopalmitate. It is important when choosing an anti-ageing product to make sure that it contains L-ascorbic acid, as this form of vitamin C has proven results when it comes to rebuilding and maintaining the dermal network.

The antioxidant effects of vitamin C are greatest when used in combination with other antioxidants such as vitamin E and ferulic acid. This may be because vitamin C is capable of regenerating oxidised vitamin E, so we get more vitamin E when the two are deployed together. It may also be that these antioxidants help prevent vitamin C-rich products from going off in the jar, ensuring its effect when eventually used on the skin.

VITAMIN E (TOCOPHEROLS AND TOCOTRIENOLS)

The term Vitamin E encompasses a family of different chemicals including tocotrienols and tocopherols. All are antioxidants. Vitamin E is widely used in cosmeceuticals to decrease skin roughness and the appearance of lines. At best it is modestly effective on its own, and only in high doses. It is more effective in preventing damage from sunlight and smoking and is a routine part of many preventive skincare regimens for these reasons. Because its dissolves in oil but not in water, vitamin E also has emollient properties and so is often used in slightly greasy moisturisers and sun creams in concentrations ranging from one percent to five percent. As noted above, it also enhances the effects of other vitamins so is often used in combination.

VITAMIN B3 (NIACIN, NICOTINIC ACID, NICOTINAMIDE OR NIACINAMIDE)

Vitamin B3 is a family of antioxidant vitamins. Niacin (also known as nicotinic acid) is converted in the body into nicotinamide, which is an essential factor in maintaining a healthy metabolism. Many cosmeceutical products contain vitamin B3 as a key antioxidant and anti-inflammatory agent. When put on the skin, vitamin B3 has been reported to improve the skin's barrier function, increase collagen production, and reduce pore size and skin blotchiness. However, these effects are modest on their own and only seen with fairly high doses (two percent to five percent).

Niacin also stimulates the circulation to increase blood flow to the skin. This can sometimes be useful, and these vitamins are often also used as 'lip plumpers' by temporarily increasing blood flow to our lips. However, changes in blood flow to the skin can be irritating for some women or cause flushing. These effects on blood flow are not seen with nicotinamide, which is stable in heat and light. However, it is more water soluble, which reduces its skin penetration abilities.

POLYPHENOLS, FLAVONOIDS AND CAROTENOIDS

Polyphenols are the largest group of chemicals found in plants. The most common polyphenols in our diet are tannins and lignins. About half of all polyphenols contain a particular kind of phenol group known as flavones, so these compounds are also called flavonoids. But as all flavonoids are polyphenols, these names are often used interchangeably in marketing. However, there are also many important non-flavonoid polyphenols including resveratrol, curcumin and ellagic acid. Some of the most popular cosmeceuticals include extracts from polyphenol-rich plants including white and green tea, rooibos, milk thistle, turmeric, soybean, chocolate, coffee berry (the unripe coffee bean), wild yam, dill seed, burdock, coral, cinnamon, rosemary, camomile, evening primrose, passion flower, aloe, ginger, gingko, lotus, peony, sage, feverfew, liquorice, rosemary, olive oil, acai berry, maci berry, endive, red orange, pomegranate, ginkgo, pine bark, and tropical ferns grapes and their seeds. It is not just one ingredient but usually a combination of chemicals that orchestrates the antioxidant effects of polyphenols. Plant extracts are also often rich in vitamins, oils, phytoestrogens and other functional chemicals that have the potential to help our skin. However, some cosmetic products contain a single purified polyphenol ingredient (like ferulic acid, ursolic acid, resveratrol, geneticin, caffeic acid, furfuryladenine or EGCG) to maximise purity and safety while minimising costs.

ALPHA LIPOIC ACID (LIPOIC ACID, THIOCTIC ACID)

Alpha lipoic acid (ALA) is a natural chemical with potent antioxidant properties. It is naturally present in our mitochondria, the cell's powerhouses. ALA has the ability to regenerate itself as well as other antioxidants like vitamins C and E, so that they can all quickly get back to neutralising free radicals. Five percent ALA is frequently added to cosmetic products along with other antioxidants. ALA is less effective as an antioxidant for the dermis, but does promote protection against sunlight damage in the epidermis.

COENZYME Q10 (COQ10 OR UBIQUINONE)

Coenzyme Q10 (CoQ10) is a key antioxidant that occurs naturally inside our skin cells. Levels of coenzyme Q10 in our skin decline from our mid-thirties onwards, and reduced levels are associated with the increased formation of free radicals. Because of this association, it makes sense to bolster our skin's CoQ10 levels and hence its defences against free radical attack. Studies have shown that topical CoQ10 can protect the skin from damage caused by sunlight; however, CoQ10 doesn't penetrate the skin very easily. To get around this, a number of different formulations have been developed, including nano-particles. The most widely used is idebenone, a synthetic analogue of CoQ10, but with better skin absorption than the natural form. Even idebenone is prone to breakdown with heat or humidity so will slowly lose some of its effectiveness once the product container is opened. People who are sensitive to chemicals like evening primrose oil may also be allergic to idebenone.

SELENIUM

Selenium is a metal ion. It is a natural constituent of some of our skin's important antioxidant enzymes. The selenium our body needs comes from our diet, mostly from eating meat, eggs and dairy products. People with low levels of selenium in their diet are more sensitive to sunlight and have an increased risk of skin cancer. It also means they have an accelerated rate of skin ageing. An obvious solution would be to put more selenium into our skin, but it is hard to get absorbed as a topical treatment. Fortunately, when combined with other chemicals (such as seleno-methionine), some selenium can be absorbed. Selenium sulphide is also used as an anti-dandruff agent and for treating itchy dermatitis, but in this form it is not significantly absorbed into the deeper layers of the skin.

MELATONIN

Melatonin is an antioxidant hormone, naturally made by our brain. Its actions in the body include regulation of our sleep-wake cycle, inflammation and immunity. Its release is disrupted by poor sleep or changing sleep cycles (see chapter 14 for more information). Melatonin is also finding its way into a number of cosmeceutical products. These mostly utilise its antioxidant properties to scavenge free radicals generated by exposure to sunlight or other noxious agents, and thereby limit the damage they cause. Like all antioxidants, it doesn't work as a remedy if applied after exposure. The radicals have already reacted and are gone. It needs to be utilised as a preventative measure. Melatonin levels are high in medicinal plants such as St. John's wort, feverfew, white and black mustard, wolfberry and fenugreek. All of these are used in various cosmetic products. Whether any of these products contain much melatonin or sufficient amounts to be effective is debatable. Melatonin and melatonin-rich plants are also used in the treatment of hair loss.

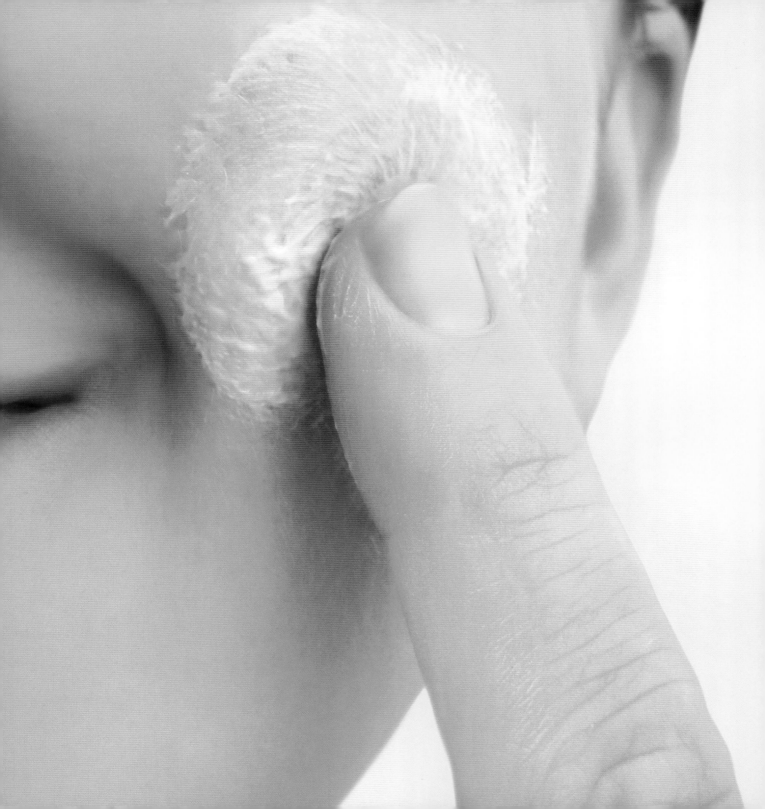

CHAPTER 20

RETINOIDS

Retinoids are a family of chemicals that are essentially relatives of vitamin A. Some retinoids are found naturally in nature and in our diet, while others are purely synthetic compounds.

They can be very effective treatments for signs of ageing and acne on the skin; however, with all retinoids there is always some potential for side effects such as irritation and flakiness. Particularly for over-the-counter retinoid treatments, the concentrations and combinations with other active ingredients can vary considerably, and so affect efficacy. Thus, it is recommended that you seek expert advice from an experienced, qualified practitioner to ensure the best course of retinoid treatment for your skin, and to monitor and adapt to any side effects that may occur.

One of the reasons for this variation in effectiveness is the many forms of retinoid that are available. One of the most well-known is retinoic acid, which was first used in the seventies for the treatment of wrinkles and acne, before research showed it could be more widely used to repair sun-damaged skin, improve fine wrinkles and mottled sun spots, and smooth the surface of the skin. Retinoic acid is a very potent form and is only available on prescription from your doctor. It is generally used after retinoid treatments with lower concentrations have been tried, as women who use this retinoid can experience redness, flaking, sensitivity to sunlight and other side effects.

The lower strength versions include retinol, retinal, and retinol palmitate (although there is little evidence that the latter improves wrinkle depth or hyperpigmentation). Because of their lower strength, these forms are less likely to irritate the skin. They can also be combined in products with other active ingredients; however, for all forms of retinoid treatments, the retinoid should not be at a concentration of more than one percent.

Retinoids are best considered as pharmaceuticals and are still the only topical agents for which there are large controlled clinical trials that support their use in the repair of damage associated with ageing and sun exposure, but they must be used with caution and taken under advisement from an expert.

Retinoic acid is naturally present in in our skin. All retinoids, natural and synthetic, either have a retinoic acid element as part of their chemical structure or get converted into retinoic acid by our skin's chemical processes. Retinoic acid repairs the skin by binding to specific receptors. This sets off a chain of chemical signals that leads to the formation of new matrix and a coordinated reduction in pathways that contribute to matrix loss, including inflammation, DNA damage and oxidative stress. This slowly stretches the skin and fills out fine wrinkles and lines, in much the same way as fillers.

By stimulating skin cell turnover, retinoids also promote the shedding of old cells and the growth of new ones in the deeper layers of the skin which then push upwards. This can improve the appearance and texture of the skin. Excess pigment production is also improved, giving the skin a more uniform appearance without the spots and blotchiness associated with ageing. Retinoids are able to significantly reverse the signs of ageing skin and restore a more youthful appearance. Retinoids may also have important effects in reducing the risk of skin cancers that are more common in ageing skin.

Although retinoids work well to restore youthful skin features, the signals that retinoids send to the skin will cease if we stop using them, and the skin starts ageing again. Skin practitioners will usually follow an initial treatment course with a long-term maintenance plan of retinoid application at a lower concentration, with lower potency retinoids or with less frequent applications.

SIDE EFFECTS OF RETINOIDS

No irritation occurs with the use of retinol palmitate; however, retinol, retinal and retinoic acid must be introduced gradually into a homecare skincare routine, as they have the potential to cause some irritation (dryness, tightness, etc.). This allows the skin cells to gain tolerance to the more active retinoids in the skin.

Retinoids are often used in the evening as exposure to UV radiation degrades their efficacy. However, retinoids can be used in the daytime as long as you use a broad spectrum sunscreen and avoid excessive exposure to sunlight. The greater the dose, the frequency, and the potency of the retinoid, the greater the risk of skin irritation.

Newer formulations and modes of application that prevent retinoids from penetrating too deep into the skin can be used to reduce the risk of skin irritation, but do not completely prevent it. Treating only once daily, or even less frequently if troublesome irritation occurs, can also reduce side effects. Some practitioners use topical anti-inflammatories or hydrocortisone creams in combination in order to reduce or prevent irritation from initial retinoid treatments. Natural compounds, such as gingko extracts, cola extract, beta-sitosterol and liquorice extract as glycyrrhetinic acid (which inhibits the cytokines that cause retinoid dermatitis) are also sometimes used in combination with retinoids to reduce skin irritation. It's also worthwhile to use an appropriate moisturiser 30 to 60 minutes after the retinoid application. However, any irritation should only be temporary when first starting to use retinoids; if irritation persists stop use and seek medical guidance. Do similarly if the skin starts to flake.

Women who are pregnant or planning to become pregnant are advised not to use retinoids, as some may have harmful effects in the developing baby (although the risk is remote as very little of the compound actually penetrates the skin).

HOW DO I KNOW IF THE RETINOL PRODUCT I CHOOSE WILL WORK?
Always ask to see results proven by images based on use of the brand's products. Clinical testing is a process that not all companies do but it is essential to be able to view before and after images. Look for retinol retinaldehyde (sometimes called retinal) on the ingredients list (although the latter is not common as it is very expensive to manufacture). These are the most effective forms. Ingredients listed as retinol palmitate or retinal acetate and retinyl-A may have anti-ageing benefits as well, although there is no conclusive clinical data. Retinoic acid is available via prescription only as it is contraindicated in pregnancy. It is prone to cause some irritation and dryness during the first few weeks of use.
CAN I DO ALL MY NORMAL ACTIVITIES IF I USE RETINOL?
Yes, but your skin will be slightly more sensitive to sunlight when using retinol, so sunscreen is a highly recommended as a precautionary measure.
WHAT IS THE BEST WAY TO START USING RETINOL?
Always start by using a low dose retinol product every other day. While most don't, some people may experience temporary skin redness or light peeling if they jump into using a retinol product daily. After you have been using it for a while and monitored your skin's reaction, increase to daily use.

CHAPTER 21
PROTEINS AND PEPTIDES

Proteins are long chains of amino acids that help specific functions in the body. Some proteins, like collagen, that help hold the skin together. Other proteins coordinate chemical reactions in the body. Some proteins regulate growth and development of our bodies.

Many cosmeceuticals contain proteins to try and trigger specific anti-ageing responses in our skin. For example, enzymes are often used as exfoliants to gently remove dead skin (see chapter 17). A number of cosmeceuticals also contain growth proteins to try to stimulate healthy skin remodelling. These are sometimes harvested from skin cells grown in a laboratory.

Peptides, however, are much shorter chains of amino acids. Peptides naturally play a role in the skin by providing chemical messages to cells, and stimulating communication between cells to prompt their functions. Peptides are much more mobile than proteins because of their small size. Peptides are found in a large number of cosmetic products and are rapidly gaining in popularity.

Our skin has its own reserves of antioxidants and it produces its own. Traditionally, skincare contains antioxidants so that it can shore up the skin reserves. However, an antioxidant peptide will theoretically instruct the skin to create more of its own antioxidants – thus getting the skin to 'think and work' for itself. For example, if too much collagen is breaking down, peptides can 'inform' the skin that it needs to make some more (KTTKS, which is a patented component of Procter & Gamble's products, performs this function). The most common reason that peptides are put into anti-ageing cosmeceuticals is to provide signals to our skin to heal the damage associated with ageing.

Human skin also contains defensive peptides (such as defensins and cathelicidins) that are released by the immune system in response to injury. Another class of peptide are fragments of proteins that work within the immune system (like antibodies, interferons, interleukins and growth factors). These assist in healing and protect against infection. Some cosmetic products aim to mimic these actions by incorporating these peptides.

Certain peptides, such as botulinum, act on nerve endings to block or enhance the signals that trigger changes in the skin. Some other peptides are able to get into the skin and inhibit key enzymes involved in matrix breakdown. This category includes peptides from wild rice, soy and even sericin, an enzyme-inhibiting peptide found in the silk produced in silkworms.

Finally, certain peptides are excellent carriers for other active ingredients and so enhance their penetration into the skin. For example, peptides are used to carry copper into the skin, an element required by some of the key enzymes involved in collagen synthesis.

The presence of active peptides in a cosmeceutical product is no guarantee that they will get into our skin in sufficient quantities or are formulated to hang around long enough to effectively do the job that we really want them to do. We know they can work, but because peptides fall under the category of cosmeceuticals, no guarantee of effectiveness is required for them to be marketed and sold. Some people claim that these often-expensive peptide products are only as good as the moisturiser in which they are dissolved. Ultimately, our choice comes down to trusting the manufacturer and then exploring how an individual product works on our skin. At least peptides are not especially irritating to the skin, as they are broken down into the same amino acids our body uses to make all our proteins.

AMINO ACIDS

Many cosmetic products claim to be high in amino acids. These are the same building blocks that comprise peptides and proteins; only they have been deconstructed into their smallest constituent elements. Most amino acids used in cosmetics are made by breaking up proteins found in soy, milk or wheat. The resulting amino acids are identical to those found in the human body. While this breakdown means they cannot perform a specific function like peptides and proteins, it doesn't mean that amino acids are without effect. In theory, by providing essential building blocks used by our skin to make protein, it might make it easier for our skin to produce matrix proteins. This is something our ageing skin doesn't do enough of. In practice, however, it is not exactly clear what amino acids do when simply put on our skin as a topical treatment. Certainly some amino acids can hang on to water so they can act as humectants (in which they are often found as an ingredient), plumping up the skin and decreasing the appearance of wrinkles. Others have wound-healing properties, while others can be combined with cell-communication ingredients for maximum benefits to the skin. Amino acids can be chemically linked to antioxidants and vitamins, which helps their penetration into the skin.

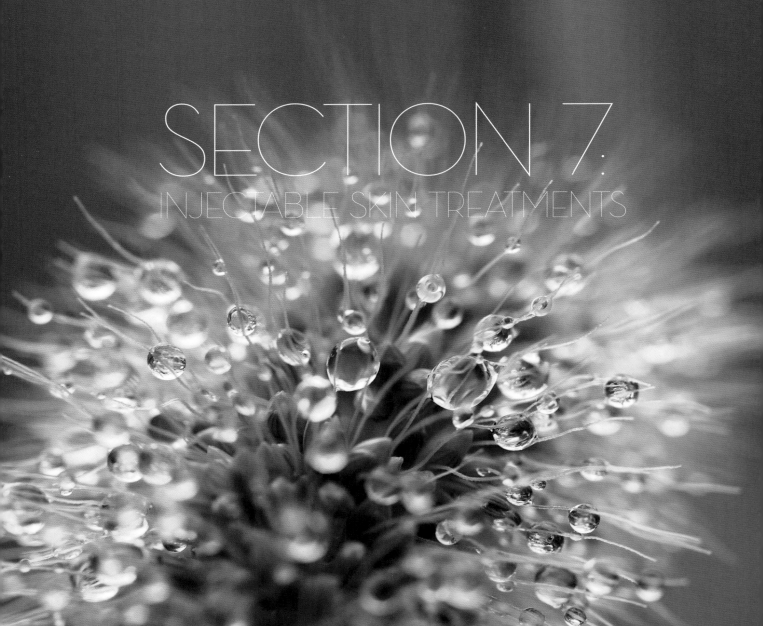

SECTION 7:
INJECTABLE SKIN TREATMENTS

CHAPTER 22: BOTULINUM NEUROTOXIN ANTI-WRINKLE INJECTIONS
CHAPTER 23: FILLERS AND VOLUMISERS
CHAPTER 24: PLATELET-RICH PLASMA (PRP)

Lines and creases occur in very specific areas on our face due to the dynamic actions of muscles that scrunch up our skin. When skin is young, it can bounce back easily, but as it gets older, the skin loses some of its elasticity. This repeated scrunching leads to deeper lines on our faces.

We also experience changes in the dermis as we age. This layer is normally thick with well-organised matrix proteins (mainly collagen, elastin and proteoglycans) that provide much of the skin's strength, elasticity and resilience, as well as some of its ability to retain water. Matrix is made by specialised skin cells known as fibroblasts, which decline in number and function as skin ages, while at the same time the delicate architecture of the dermis becomes disorganised and dysfunctional. With the redistribution of fat and a reduction in moisture content, our skin sags, hollows and wrinkles without the strength of the elastic dermis to hold it tight.

To combat this, one simple method is to temporarily weaken or paralyse the muscles that produce the wrinkles on our face. This is achieved by injecting specific muscles with chemicals that block the signals coming from nerves that tell them to contract. There are a number of anti-wrinkle injections on the market. Practitioners have their preferences but it's best not to simply go on the brand name, or the price. If you pay peanuts, you might get a monkey! The best practitioners know the muscles intimately and are artists when it comes to injecting in just the right spot to get a challenging muscle to lift.

To correct the loss of tissue and prevent its sagging we can inject substances into or under our skin. The aim is to fill out any deep wrinkles, folds and creases, to smooth out the skin and restore an appearance of youthful fullness. This is called soft tissue augmentation. This technique is often used on breasts, but also works effectively for sagging skin and hollowed angular contours on other parts of the body – in expert hands, it can also be used for facial sculpting or contouring, to augment the shape of the jaw line or cheeks.

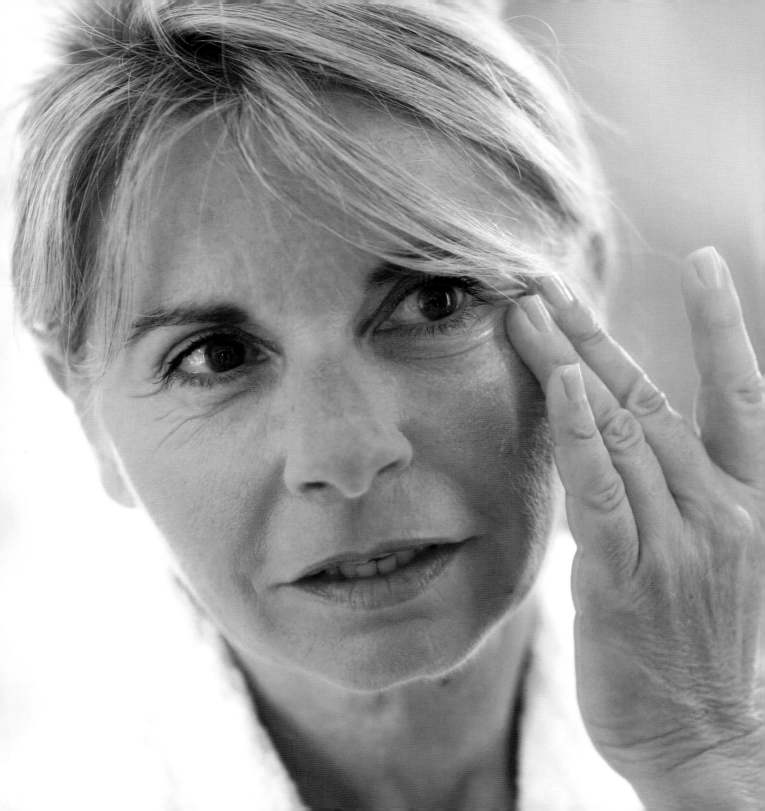

CHAPTER 22:

BOTULINUM NEUROTOXIN ANTI-WRINKLE INJECTIONS

Anti-wrinkle injections have long been known as 'botox' therapy; however, Botox® is a brand name and just one of several effective formulations of nerve blocking agents available. Other similar products include Dysport® and Xeomin®.

All of these products contain the muscle-paralysing chemical found in a bacterium called clostridium botulinum, which is a neurotoxin. Researchers in the 1960s discovered that injecting tiny quantities of type A botulinum toxin into overactive muscles could cause a temporary paralysis that lasted for a period of three to four months. It quickly became a useful treatment for a diverse range of conditions in which overactivity of one particular muscle was a problem, including crossed or lazy eyes (strabismus), uncontrollable blinking (blepharospasm) and involuntary contractions of neck muscles (cervical dystonia).

In the late 1980s, it became clear that these injections were also a valuable treatment for wrinkles produced by contracting muscles in the face. Since then it has become the most frequently used and widespread of all procedures in cosmetic medicine, and is often used as the first-line treatment for facial wrinkles and lines. In expert hands, injections are easy to administer and can achieve consistent and fast results with minimal complication. Currently, over half a million procedures are performed annually in Australia alone.

HOW DO ANTI-WRINKLE INJECTIONS WORK?

The main reason for getting these injections is to smooth out unsightly lines, creases and wrinkles in our face. They work because the muscles that pull the lines onto our face are relaxed or paralysed by the toxin, meaning the wrinkle line can't form. The botulinum toxin works to block the chemical signals that trigger muscular contractions. In low doses the muscle is simply relaxed, while in higher doses it is completely paralysed. These injections don't damage the muscle or the nerve, but essentially just put the muscle to sleep. With fewer muscle contractions, the overlying skin progressively smooths out and fine wrinkles soften to restore a more youthful and relaxed appearance. The final result is similar to how the wrinkle looks when we are asleep, when the muscle is fully relaxed.

These injections do not work, however, for static wrinkles (also known as resting lines) that are prominent even when the face is relaxed or we are asleep; blocking the muscle contraction will not take them away. Static wrinkles are generally treated with fillers or facelifts.

The injections are delivered precisely into specific muscles, so any areas that are not injected will still function normally, allowing the muscles to contract with natural expressions such as smiling. This is unless we accidentally rub the area to spread the dose or our practitioner is not precise with injections or dosing. In such cases, which are very uncommon, some adjacent muscles may be affected, as the toxin diffuses out of the target area.

While injecting botulinum toxin is a straightforward procedure and can be performed by many different practitioners, there are many complex differences in our faces. Expertise is required in facial anatomy, but also the skin's responses to different doses. It should always be delivered by a trained, licensed health professional.

Although it is effective on its own, neurotoxin injections are increasingly used in combination with other cosmetic procedures, including fillers, resurfacing, IPL and cosmetic surgery. It is thought that such combinations may be complementary and synergistic to achieve a more polished, refined and longer-lasting result.

WHO SHOULDN'T HAVE ANTI-WRINKLE INJECTIONS?

Some medications, including antihypertensive calcium-channel blockers, quinine (for cramps), aminoglycoside antibiotics, and penicillamine (for Wilson's disease), can impact upon the effects of botulinum toxin and may need to be stopped before undertaking the procedure. Botulinum toxins should not be administered to women who are either pregnant or nursing. (Women who were treated during pregnancy have had normal babies; however, this does not rule out the potential for harm.)

PREPARATION FOR ANTI-WRINKLE INJECTIONS

It is typical for photographs to be taken before all cosmetic procedures, in order to evaluate the results. This is especially important for botulinum toxin injections, with photos taken both at rest and with the muscles contracted (i.e. frowning or smiling) to assess what has been achieved and decide whether there is a need for further treatment. The best timing for the procedure will depend on the overall cosmetic treatment plan. When it is combined with other treatments, such as laser resurfacing or facelifts, some practitioners prefer to inject in the post-operative period.

Minimal preparation is needed before the procedure. Your practitioner may ask you to avoid taking warfarin, aspirin or anti-inflammatory drugs like NSAIDS (e.g. ibuprofen, ketoprofen) one to two weeks before the procedure to reduce the risk of bruising. Some practitioners also recommend stopping vitamin E, ginseng, fish-oil tablets, or herbal supplements with blood-thinning effects for the same reason. On the day of your treatment, make sure that your skin is free from any facial products, such as makeup, moisturiser, lotion and oil.

ANTI-WRINKLE INJECTION PROCEDURE

Injections should be performed by a qualified medical practitioner or by a registered nurse who is supervised by a medical practitioner. You should always be treated sitting up on a bed, not lying down. Before the injection, the area for treatment is thoroughly cleansed with an antiseptic agent and then dried. Then the practitioner will mark the target areas for injection symmetrically on both sides of the face. This is important to keep the natural balance of our face. The practitioner will usually select three to five injection points for each area to be treated.

Choosing the right dose is as critical as choosing the site of injection. Depending on the technique, the severity of wrinkles, their location, and the activity and size of the target muscle, the dose per injection will range from five to fifty units with Botox® and Xeomin®, while the dose required for Dysport® is two and a half times higher. The full dose is then divided into equal parts across all injection sites. There are well-established dosing protocols for treating different issues, but the best guide is the experience of the practitioner.

Although there is little difference between the products in terms of their effectiveness, some studies have shown that Dysport® works a little more quickly than Botox®, but it may also show greater diffusion and migration into adjacent muscles.

The procedure itself is almost painless because of the fine calibre of the needles and the tiny volumes that are used. Painkillers are not necessary; however, some practitioners and patients prefer that a local anaesthesia or numbing cream be applied before the procedure. Some practitioners also apply ice to partially numb an area and reduce any potential bruising, swelling and redness.

After the procedure, don't touch the area for at least four hours. You should be able to go about your normal daily routine immediately; however, very vigorous activities should be avoided for 24 hours after the procedure. This will maximise the effects in the target area and reduce unwanted effects on other muscles.

HOW LONG WILL ANTI-WRINKLE INJECTIONS LAST?

The advent of botulinum toxin injections has been one of the most important advances for the treatment of ageing skin. When used appropriately they can almost always produce improvements in the signs of ageing. Most women undergoing the procedure come away feeling satisfied with the result.

The effects may not be immediately obvious after the injection. It is normal to have to wait for three to five days before any improvement of wrinkles is noticed, but the best effects tend to be achieved after one to two weeks. So don't rush into getting a re-treatment if the results are not immediately apparent.

Remember that the effects of each injection are only temporary. The muscle that has been partly or completely paralysed by the injection gradually regains its ability to contract. Botulinum normally lasts three to four months, with some people achieving five to six months. Its effect is often influenced by your metabolism and whether you've had the treatment in conjunction with other cosmetic procedures aimed at the prevention of wrinkles, like fillers, laser or retinoids.

RISKS OF ANTI-WRINKLE INJECTIONS

The use of botulinum toxin for the treatment of wrinkles is well established throughout the world. For the many millions of treatments performed globally it has an excellent safety profile. This does not mean that it is always without complications. We have all seen or heard of stories of something going wrong, but rest assured, serious complications are rare.

The most common adverse effects reported are mild, local and transitory. These include redness, bruising, swelling, pain and an increase in sensitivity around the injection site. In most cases this is due to technical issues such as the choice of dose, the injection site and the skill of the practitioner delivering it. Some people also report fatigue, malaise, flu-like symptoms, nausea and rashes at sites distant from the injection area, which are usually treated symptomatically (for example, with painkillers for headache) and tend to settle quickly.

In some cases, injections may inadvertently cause muscle weakness outside of the target area. For example, treatment of lines above the eyes occasionally causes a temporary drooping of the upper eyelid (known as ptosis). Ptosis may occur as early as 48 hours after the procedure or as late as seven to ten days after an injection. Injections on forehead creases may cause temporary drooping of the eyebrows (known as brow ptosis) creating a 'cockeyed' appearance. Treatment of crow's feet may sometimes cause double vision (known as diplopia), turning out of the lower eyelid and an asymmetric smile. This site is also especially prone to bruising following an injection. In a few instance, the botulinum can move beyond the site of the injection and cause discomfort in non-target areas.

To reduce the risk of these complications, a practitioner will always try to accurately inject the lowest effective dose in the smallest volume (the highest concentration), so that any migration of effects into areas that were not targeted during the procedure will be minimised. Dividing treatment sessions may also be useful if a large number of injections are required. To maximise potential benefits while minimising potential harm, each procedure must be carefully administered at the right dose, in the right location and at the correct time intervals. It is also important not to use the treatment too often, as this can lead to muscle thinning and atrophy. Assessing muscle movement and strength in the area to be injected is also important and can avoid potential side effects such as ptosis.

SIDE EFFECTS OF ANTI-WRINKLE INJECTIONS

If an area of treated skin is exposed to very cold temperatures, some women experience bruising and/or swelling as blood returns to the treated area as it subsequently warms. Swelling is more common in areas with lots of blood flow, such as around the eyes and lips. This can be reduced by applying steroid cream immediately after the procedure.

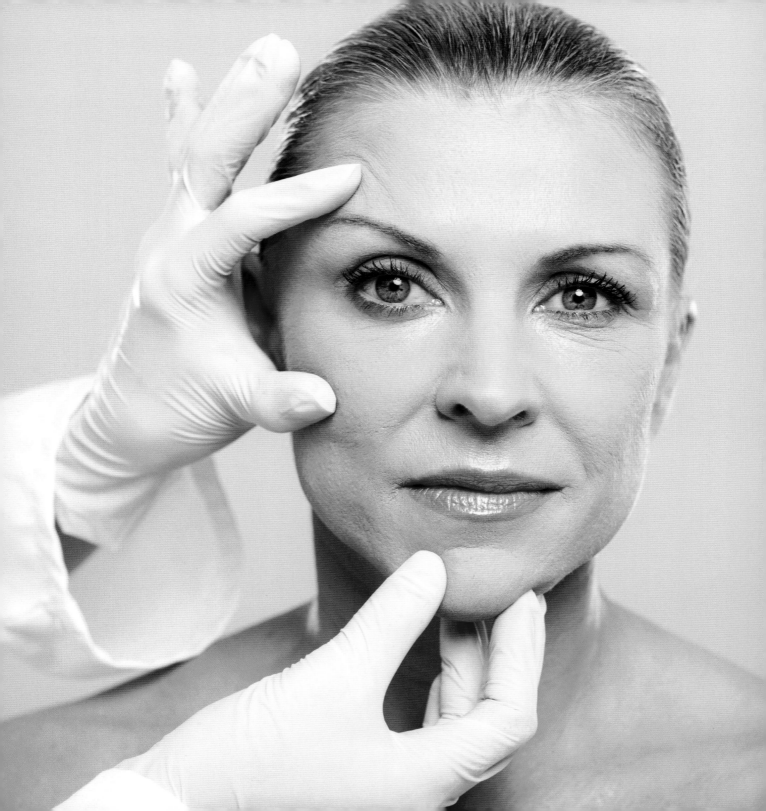

CHAPTER 23

FILLERS AND VOLUMISERS

Filler injections work by drawing in water to the skin and holding it there as a means to bulk up the skin in a particular target area. The filling effect of these injections is immediate; however, their cosmetic effect only lasts as long as it takes for our body to break down and absorb the injected material. Today many fillers achieve 12 to 18 months' longevity. This varies from product to product, but all fillers must be reinjected at regular intervals to maintain their effect.

Some injected substances aim to directly stimulate the production of natural matrix-bulking components in the skin. These agents are known as volumisers. Unlike fillers, the full effect of volumisers may take some weeks to evolve, as new dermal matrix is progressively generated and laid down through a series of treatments. However, their cosmetic effect can last for many years, as the rate of turnover of collagen in the skin is slow. Volumisers generally don't need to be frequently reapplied, although touch-ups are sometimes needed to maintain an optimal result. Many cosmetic injections combine both fillers and volumisers in a single product, to get an instant and long-lasting result in which the volume of new matrix production slowly replaces the filler.

There are many different products available. Each has its own specific properties that make it suitable for certain uses in different parts of the face and at different times. Safety, durability and versatility also vary from product to product. The choice of which agent or combination of agents will be best for your particular skin and its needs is crucial in order to achieve the desired outcomes and to avoid potential complications.

INJECTABLE COLLAGEN

Injectable collagens (such as Zyderm and Zyplast) were among the first fillers to be used in cosmetic medicine. Collagen is a matrix protein that is a major structural component of the dermis of the skin. The amount and quality of collagen in our skin declines as we get older. The point of injecting collagen is to do the same job as our own collagen, which is to provide structure, elasticity, flexibility and volume, and thus improve the appearance. Once injected, the collagen immediately makes that area of the skin fuller. This filling effect is temporary and lasts for between three and nine months as the body slowly absorbs the injected collagen. For optimal results, repeated treatments of two to four injections are usually necessary when using collagen on its own. Collagen is often combined with hyaluronic acid (HA) or other volumisers to maximise the initial effect on the skin's appearance and at the same time stimulate matrix production for longer lasting results.

HYALURONIC ACID

Hyaluronic acid (HA) products (such as brands such as Juvaderm, Restylane, Emervel and Perlane) are among the most popular injectable fillers. Products containing HA now comprise at least three out of every four skin augmentation procedures. HA is a natural component of the skin, so does not cause allergic reactions. It is a glycosaminoglycan (GAG) that attracts and holds water, which serves to plump up the skin. Young skin is full of moisture and volume, due in part to the abundance of HA and other GAGs. As we age, the production of GAGs in the skin declines. This results in a loss of skin hydration, volume and elasticity, contributing to wrinkling, sagging and the hollowing out of facial features. Because HA keeps the skin hydrated, it has also become a popular ingredient in many skincare products, although its penetration is limited when used in a topical cream.

HAs can be extracted from animal tissue (for example, rooster combs) or produced using bacteria. In our skin, HA is rapidly turned over every few days, so injecting straight HA would not be of value. However, the hydrating properties of HA can be harnessed in fillers, by chemically cross-linking a large number of HA molecules together. This transforms liquid HA into a gel, which can then be injected. The injected HA adds volume to the skin as it absorbs more than 1000 times its own weight in water. The chemical cross-linking of HA also slows its breakdown, prolonging its effectiveness within the skin. The more cross-linked the product, the longer its effect will be, but it will never be permanent. The downside is that these highly cross-linked agents are more challenging to place correctly, compared with other fillers, because of their thicker viscosity. However, a key advantage of HA is that any excessive filling or filling in the wrong place can be quickly reversed with an injection of hyaluronidase, a natural enzyme that breaks down HA.

POLYLACTIC ACID

Polylactic acid (PLA) (found in brands such as Sculptra®) is a synthetic polymer of lactic acid that is fully biodegradable. PLA has been used since the 1960s in dissolvable sutures. In cosmetic procedures, PLA is primarily used as a facial volumiser, especially on the temples, cheeks and mid-face. It is becoming more widely used as an all-purpose filler and shaper to re-contour an ageing face. Each injection is made up of thousands of polylactic acid beads (known as microparticles). When first injected, these beads fill the wrinkles only slightly, with the main volumising effect coming from the carrier fluid that is injected into the area at the same time. However, over subsequent weeks and months, the PLA stimulates the skin's production of collagen by triggering the body's natural healing response. The matrix of collagen and elastic fibres, which are laid down from the skin's reaction to the PLA beads, steadily increases the volume of the injected areas of skin, smoothing out depressions and strengthening the skin's structure and the facial tissues underneath.

A series of treatments (usually three or four) performed a month apart are usually required to achieve full re-contouring of the face. This ensures a smooth and natural looking appearance. Due to the very slow breakdown of PLA (into lactate, a chemical found naturally in the human body), and the prolonged stimulation of collagen production, PLA's effects as a volumiser are long-lasting, in most cases for at least two to three years after the end of the treatment.

CALCIUM HYDROXYLAPATITE

Calcium hydroxylapatite (found in brands such as Radiesse®) is a synthetic volumiser that is popular for the treatment of wrinkles, folds, facial fat loss, nose bumps and skin hollowness. It is also widely used in bone health supplements, as it is a good source of calcium. However, when taken orally, it has no effect on skin tone or wrinkles.

Calcium hydroxylapatite was one of the first volumisers. It is a naturally occurring mineral component of bone and teeth (so there is no chance of allergy). When injected into the skin, microparticles stimulate the skin to make collagen and act as a scaffold to hold it in place. This new collagen slowly fills out the injected area, making the skin look and feel more plump, smoothing out wrinkles and facial folds, and restoring a youthful appearance. The calcium microparticles are only slowly broken down by the body, which accounts for the prolonged effect of these volumisers. Although good results can be achieved after one treatment, additional touch-ups are sometimes needed. The effects of one injection series will, in most cases, last for about one to two years after the end of the treatment period, depending on age, skin type and lifestyle.

POLYACRYLAMIDE GEL

Polyacrylamide gel (found in brands such as Aquamid®) is a permanent filler made up from 97–98 percent water and 2–3 percent cross-linked polyacrylamide. This forms a soft hydrogel that, in contrast to PLA, does not contain any microparticles. It is injected under the skin into the subdermis, where it can't be broken down. In essence, this is a small-scale injectable implant which performs a similar role to breast implants –

permanently augmenting soft tissue. Because the hydrogel is very elastic it moves naturally with all facial expressions. Different permanent fillers are available in countries other than Australia, such as including polymethyl methacrylate (in brands like ArteFill®) and expanded polytetrafluoroethylene (e-PTFE; also known as Teflon®).

WHAT HAPPENS DURING THE PROCEDURE?

Injection with dermal fillers is a simple procedure and there is usually no downtime required for recovery, so you can return to your normal activities immediately. It is advisable, however, to avoid prolonged exposure to the sun, heat or cold, and to refrain from doing strenuous physical activities for a day or two after the treatment, as these can increase the risk of bruising and swelling. It is also important not to touch the injected areas, and to minimise exaggerated facial expressions for a day or two. It is also recommended not to use makeup for a day or so, not because it is bad for the skin, but because you don't really want any excess pressure on the injection sites.

With volumisers it is recommended to do the opposite and frequently massage the treated areas for a week or so post-treatment in order to prevent the formation of lumps or an uneven appearance.

Injections with filler or volumiser are a medical procedure that should only be performed by a licensed practitioner at the practitioner's office or private clinic. Preparation is minimal. You should avoid taking warfarin, aspirin or anti-inflammatory drugs, like NSAIDS (e.g. ibuprofen, ketoprofen) one to two weeks before the procedure in order to reduce the risk of bruising. Some practitioners also recommend stopping vitamin E, ginseng, fish-oil tablets, or herbal supplements with anticoagulant effects for the same reason.

After the practitioner's assessment, the face is washed with soap and water or with an antiseptic, and then insertion points are marked with a non-permanent pen. Although the treatment is not painful, the practitioner may inject a mild localised anaesthetic or apply a topical numbing cream on the target areas prior to injection, to help reduce any feelings of discomfort. Putting ice or cold compresses on the skin before, during and after the injections, is another method that can be used to improve comfort and reduce bruising.

During the procedure, the skin is held taut by the practitioner's hand and a fine needle is carefully introduced at an angle parallel to the skin for superficial lines and wrinkles, and at a steeper angle for deeper lines and grooves. A series of small injections are made, along or adjacent to the wrinkle being treated. Each treatment takes approximately 15 to 30 minutes, depending on the number of areas to be injected.

It is common to receive injections over two or three sessions, each about a month apart, to ensure full coverage of an area and to get the best results.

AREAS THAT CAN BE TREATED WITH DERMAL FILLERS

> Temples
> Cheeks
> Lips
> Hands
> Most areas in the face

POSSIBLE SIDE EFFECTS OF FILLER INJECTIONS

Any injection into the face, even with tiny needles, can cause some bruising, swelling, redness or tenderness at the injection site. This is common and often inevitable. These side effects usually disappear after a few days, but if they persist or get worse contact the practitioner and seek medical advice.

Some patients receiving filler may experience small lumps or nodules, most commonly at the injection sites. If the injection is too superficial, it may lead to visible white, yellow, or blue nodules, which may be persistent in some cases. Injections too deep below the skin can mean the procedure doesn't work as well as expected, and may need to be repeated. Any issues should always be followed up with your practitioner, as there are often some simple corrective actions that can be undertaken. Such side effects are typically the result of the injection process itself, and are less common with experienced practitioners.

Nodules are not a problem with volumisers as they do not create as much bulk as fillers. Volumisers should not be used for lip or breast augmentation or on areas close to the eyes. Neither fillers nor volumisers should be administered to pregnant women or those nursing. Volumisers should also not be used if you have a susceptibility to bad scarring (keloid or hypertrophic scarring). With the exception of animal collagens, fillers are not associated with allergic reactions, although all may be temporarily irritating to the skin. An allergy skin test can be useful prior to the treatment for those using products containing animal collagen.

Some laboratories grow autologous cells in serum obtained from the calves on your legs. This means that there remains a potential for an allergic reaction even though these cells are derived from human skin. The issue of cancer has been raised with this autologous cell therapy. By encouraging cells to grow, it is proposed that any cancerous cells in the body might grow uncontrollably. However, to date there has been no evidence for this, and it is fully approved as a safe treatment in many countries.

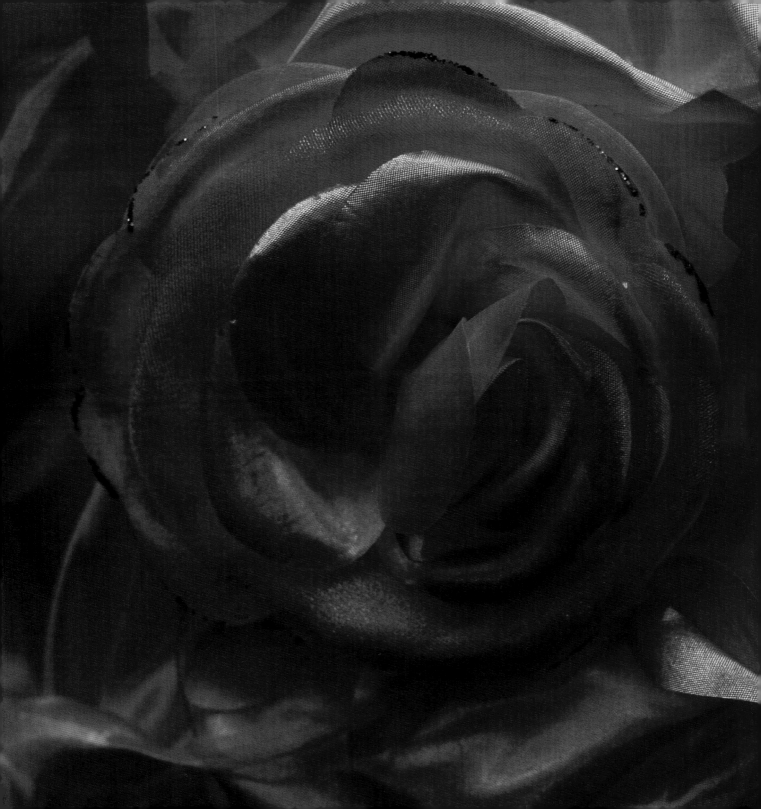

CHAPTER 24

PLATELET-RICH PLASMA (PRP)

Platelet-rich plasma (PRP) has been a successful part of sports medicine for a number of years. The key to its success is the high concentration of platelets, an agent in blood that promotes repair to damaged cells. In fact, the number of platelets in this plasma product is usually between five and ten times higher than that normally found in blood. This is important when it comes to creating healthy skin as these platelets are the key to any kind of tissue repair in the body.

The concentrated platelets in PRP contain large quantities of bioactive proteins known as growth factors. These growth factors are pivotal in the repair and regeneration of the skin. They initiate connective tissue repair and improve overall wound healing. You see them at work any time that you cut yourself; the platelets are what cause the blood to clot. This is a natural defence that the body uses when it needs to heal itself. In addition, the platelets in PRP encourage collagen production and attract more stem cells to damaged area, which helps the body to heal and produce new cells. The result is an improvement in skin texture and quality, including a thicker upper epidermal layer. The plasma is generated from the patient's own blood, ensuring compatibility and mitigating disease transmission or allergic reaction.

PRP is often used in combination with other treatments to improve tissue regeneration and rejuvenation, to increase collagen production and to aid healing and reduce downtime. For instance, it is often used in conjunction with a radio frequency treatment, as the two promote healthy collagen growth in different ways. Furthermore, when combined with anti-wrinkle injections and dermal fillers, PRP treatments can make significant improvements to difficult-to-treat areas such as around the eyes or mouth.

WHAT HAPPENS DURING THE PROCEDURE?

A small amount of blood is extracted, generally from the arm. This is no more than 10–20 millilitres and will be collected in a special sterile tube. This blood will be placed in a centrifuge for 5–8 minutes in order to separate the plasma and concentrate the platelets.

The platelets are extracted and injected into the deeper layers of the skin to increase collagen synthesis, resulting in an increase in improvements in skin thickness, tightness and overall health. Depending on the area to be treated the PRP can either be administered to the skin during a skin needling procedure or injected directly under the skin when a more precise application is required. In addition, PRP can be applied to the skin following a fractionated laser treatment to shorten the downtime and improve results.

For the best results it is recommended that the treatment be comprised of a series of injections spread out over several weeks. Generally, three treatments performed once every 4–5 weeks will give the best outcome. Results generally take time and many people experience continued improvements for one or two years after the end of the treatment period.

AREAS THAT CAN BE TREATED WITH PRP

> **Around the eyes.** This delicate area will require a series of injections with fine needles to facilitate tightening of the skin and reduce the appearance of tiny wrinkles and loose skin. The fine needles will facilitate precise targeting of the PRP for optimal results.
> **Cheeks and mid face.** As we age, these areas tend to sag as the skin grows loose. Practitioners often use a Dermastamp device that has multiple tiny needles so that injections can be applied evenly across the area to give a uniform result.
> **Neck and décolletage.** These can become problem areas when the combination of gravity and loose skin results in what is often termed 'chicken neck'. A Dermastamp approach is often used for this area, not only giving a uniform result but also allowing a larger area to be treated in a shorter amount of time.
> **Jaw line.** Most of us experience a drooping or softening of the jaw line with age, caused by the skin losing its elasticity, along with the long-term effects of gravity. This can be countered with an injection of PRP using fine needles along the jaw line.
> **Back of hands.** It is not uncommon to see a skeletisation of the hands, particularly on the backs, as we age. Because the hands are the one part of our body that is almost constantly exposed to the rays of the sun, they also tend to have the most sun damage. Even if you remember to put sunscreen on your hands, chances are it will be rubbed or washed off. The skin on the back of our hands becomes thin and damaged due to a loss of the collagen and

elastin fibres that give it the smooth texture. Another side effect of all that sun on our hands is solar lentigos, commonly called sun spots or age spots. The combination of bony hands, thin skin and dark age spots makes many of us feel our hands look older than they should. The typical PRP treatment for hands is relatively quick, taking between 20 minutes and a half hour to complete.

> **Scalp (to reduce hair loss).** While male pattern baldness is a common problem for many men, women can also experience some degree of hair loss as they age, particularly around the crown. PRP treatments can help to reduce the amount of hair loss. The increased level of platelets encourages the growth of new blood vessels, giving hair follicles a richer blood supply. This can also rejuvenate dormant hair follicles and thus create a richer and thicker head of hair.

POSSIBLE SIDE EFFECTS OF PRP INJECTIONS

Immediately after PRP injections some people complain about a mild ache or soreness at the site of the injections. You can expect some amount of redness and tenderness in the area for the next day or two. In some cases, this can be accompanied by a small amount of bruising. However, this usually only takes a few days to resolve itself, and depends on how prone individual patients are to bruising. Patients may also experience a few days of minor swelling after PRP injections.

AFTERCARE

Following PRP injections there is no specific aftercare other than to keep the injection sites clean and to drink plenty of water to ensure that the body is well hydrated. After PRP is applied it is beneficial not to wash the application area for 24 hours in order to allow the growth factors to penetrate into the skin and stimulate healing. Applying a silicon layer after PRP assists in locking in the beneficial growth factors.

STEM CELL THERAPY

Stem cell therapy is a relatively new technique to add volume and/or reduce wrinkles and sagging in the skin on the face. Stem cells are elements in our body that stimulate other cells into action – in this case tightening the skin, renewing skin cells and improving collagen production. Unlike a surgical facelift, which lifts and repositions tissues, stem cell therapy simply helps the skin rejuvenate itself.

Because everyone's stem cells are unique, the procedure needs to extract stem cells from one part of your body in order to add them to your face. If stem cells from someone else were used, your body would treat them as foreign bodies and destroy them.

And don't worry; adding stem cells won't mean you grow an extra nose on your face or anything. Because the stem cells respond to and stimulate the cells around them, if they are added to the face they will only cause natural facial processes to occur.

What effects does stem cell therapy have?

Often a stem cell therapy is used to add volume to the skin on the face. This involves combining the stem cells with fat for injection into specific targeted areas. If, however, you are just trying to achieve a tighter, more youthful texture to the skin, rather than adding volume, the stem cells alone are used. In both cases, you should see visibly younger looking skin soon after the treatment.

What to expect during the procedure?

There are two parts to the stem cell therapy treatment, requiring two separate visits to the clinic. The first procedure is to extract the stem cells. They are typically taken from the abdomen or the upper part of the buttocks. The practitioner applies a local anaesthetic to numb the area, and then uses a needle to extract the fat.

The fat is then sent to the laboratory to separate the stem cells from the fat. This typically takes a couple of weeks, as the sample is checked for infections and the stem cells are checked for viability (it is recommended that you choose a practitioner whose process involves manually checking the viability of the stem cells – automated checks have been known to return false results). The stem cells are then stimulated to increase in number in the laboratory.

Once sufficient stem cells have been produced, you return to the clinic and the cells are injected into the target areas of your face. Whether being applied with fat or not, the cells are combined with a little PRP for ease of delivery. It is then injected into the skin.

What to expect after the procedure?

Following the treatment, your face may feel somewhat stingy, and it can experience redness and tenderness for a few days. There can also be some minimal pinpoint bleeding from the injection sites, but this will usually settle within 24 hours. Occasionally you may notice excessive swelling or bruising, but this is usually the result of an inexperienced practitioner, and can be easily remedied. Follow your normal skincare regimen. You should notice improvements in skin volume/texture within two to three days of the procedure, as any inflammation subsides. Because stem cell therapy is a relatively recent addition to facial skincare, there are no long term studies on its effects, but practitioners suggest that the effects could last for between five and eight years.

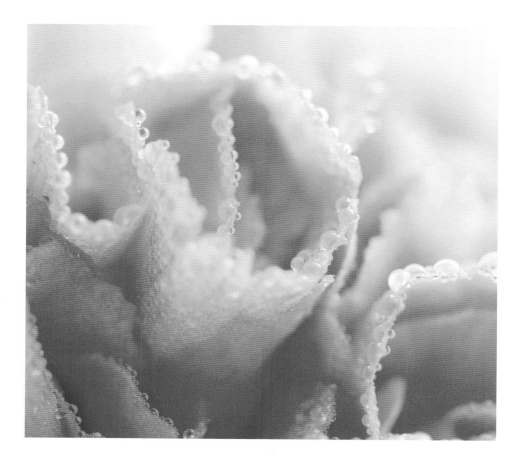

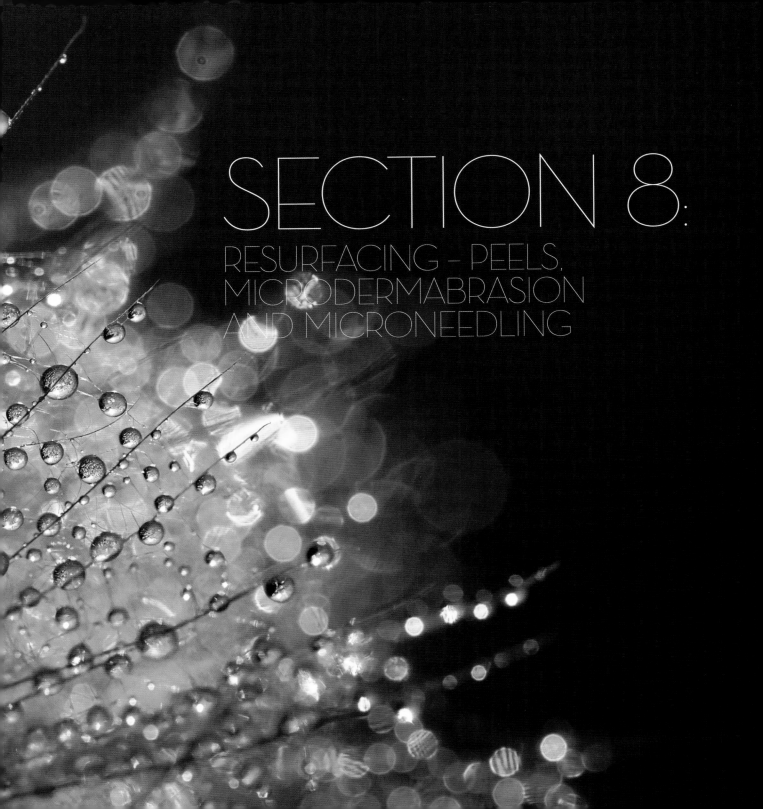

SECTION 8:
RESURFACING – PEELS, MICRODERMABRASION AND MICRONEEDLING

CHAPTER 25: CHEMICAL PEELS
CHAPTER 26: MICRODERMABRASION
CHAPTER 27: MICRONEEDLING

Resurfacing does two important things to the appearance of the skin. Firstly, the skin immediately looks younger as newer, plumper skin cells are now visible. Secondly, the skin will increase the production of new skin cells to make up for the sudden shortfall from the surface, which further aids the shedding of the dead, outer skin cells. The only problem is that the effects of resurfacing are short lived. Once skin thickness is restored, old skin often goes back to its sluggish ways. This is one reason why many skin creams include exfoliants, which act to promote skin turnover by helping the shedding of old skin.

There are a number of ways to resurface the skin and in this section we look at three of them: chemical peels, microdermabrasion and microneedling.

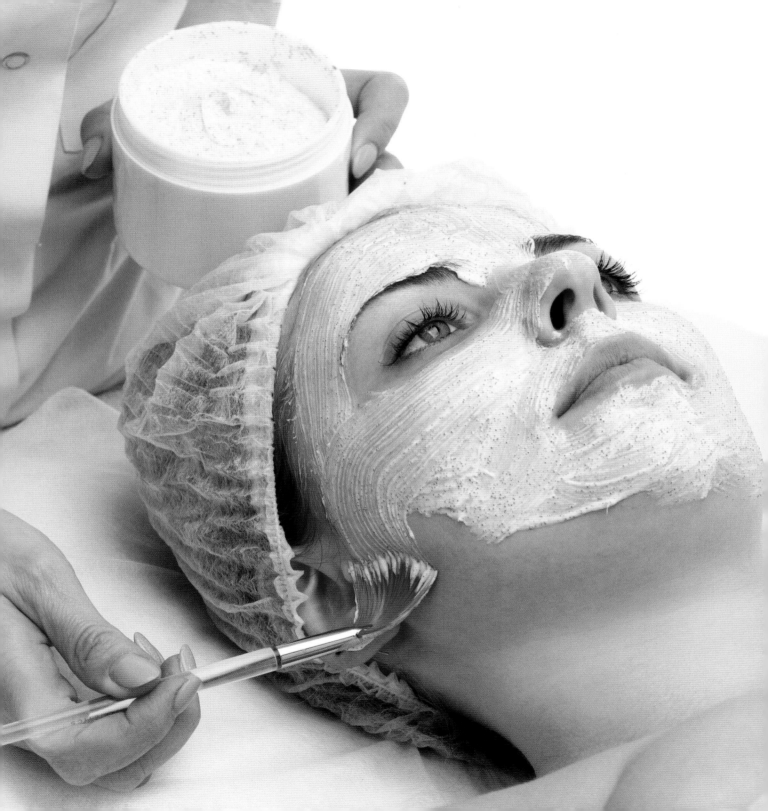

CHAPTER 25:
CHEMICAL PEELS

A chemical peel is one of the most popular and quickest ways to remove the outer layers of our skin. It is also known as exfoliation, resurfacing or refreshing. Women have used chemical peels for skin rejuvenation for centuries.

Chemical peels treat and improve the appearance of age spots, fine wrinkles, acne, uneven skin pigmentation and sun damage, primarily on the face but also on the décolletage, neck, back and hands. Peels can also be used to treat 'chicken skin' on the back, legs, buttocks and arms. Chemical peels are not generally recommended for the treatment of sagging skin, lumps or severe wrinkles, and they should not be used on the eyelids.

Chemical peels use one or more chemicals (known as exfoliants) to remove varying amounts of the dead cells that comprise the outer layers of the skin. These chemicals are usually acids or organic solvents.

All chemical peels work in much the same way, wounding the skin and breaking down the connections between cells to allow dead cells on the surface of the skin to be shed. New skin cells can then emerge to replace the old and damaged skin, improving skin texture, colour and appearance.

Chemical peels can be broadly classified into superficial, medium and deep peels, with the classification being determined by the depth of a peel, the concentration and strength of the chemical in the peel, and its time in contact with the skin.

The type of peel we need depends on our particular skin problem, our skin type and tolerance to chemicals. Different types of peel also have different application requirements. Deep procedures should only be performed by experienced physicians, while superficial peels can often be performed in the comfort of your own home.

SUPERFICIAL PEELS

Normally the dead layer of cells covering the outer surface of the skin protects the underlying living skin cells from harm. This changes after a superficial peel, as with the removal of dead skin cells from the surface, living skin cells are exposed to the outside world. This accelerates the normal process of exfoliation; so younger, plumper cells now sit on the surface. Live skin cells react to being on the surface by sending messages to the underlying skin make more new skin cells and a stronger skin matrix. Their greater moisture content makes the skin look and feel younger and smoother. Superficial peels are often used in combination with topical treatments because they are not required to penetrate deep into the skin.

Superficial peels are a good starting point for exploring cosmeceuticals. Healing is rapid, with little downtime; they are relatively low cost and have few potential side effects. However, their benefits are relatively short-term. This means superficial peels are generally repeated every one to four weeks in a series of three to six treatments until the desired results are achieved. Yet even then the skin will generally return to its previous state within one to two years after the treatment has ended (although the use of complementary topical agents can extend this time). This is also why, for the best, longest lasting results, superficial chemical peels are often used in combination with other rejuvenating and resurfacing techniques.

It is a common misconception that a series of several superficial peels will produce the same result as one deeper peel. In fact, as they target different layers of the skin, they can have very different effects. For example, superficial peels, even if repeated again and again, will never succeed in treating deep wrinkles.

A superficial peel uses low concentrations of weak acids, such as 10–25 percent trichloroacetic acid (TCA), 20–30 percent salicylic acid (BHA) or alpha-hydroxy acid (AHA), 20–30 percent glycolic acid, 30 percent lactic acid or 40 percent mandelic acid. There are also superficial peels that use enzymes, such as bromelain and 1 percent retinol, which are painless and effective. Many of these acids are found in nature, such as in sugar cane, sour milk or citrus; however, all acids used in superficial peels are now specifically manufactured to ensure purity. Gone are the days of using lemon juice!

WHAT HAPPENS DURING THE PROCEDURE?

Once placed on the skin these acids will keep working until they are neutralised (by a basic solution) and/or washed away. It takes some experience to judge the right moment to stop the procedure. Neutralise too early and you get poorer results, but neutralise too late and you may end up with more redness or other side effects. Partially neutralised and self-neutralising peels are sometimes used to mitigate this requirement. Trichloroacetic acid (TCA) can't be easily neutralised, so the concentration and total amount of TCA that is applied to the skin has to be perfectly calculated and perfectly applied to get an even response.

MEDIUM AND DEEP PEELS

Medium and deep peels are used to treat more significant skin irregularities, such as hyperpigmentation, deep wrinkles and long-term sun damage. To achieve the full effect, the peel must penetrate as deep as the deepest skin problem. The deeper the peel, the more long-lasting the benefits. However, this does not mean that a deeper treatment will necessarily yield a more effective result. It all depends on the symptom being treated, and deeper peels do have a greater potential for side effects, including redness, swelling and hyper- or even hypopigmentation.

A medium peel uses trichloroacetic acid (TCA) in concentrations of 35 percent to 50 percent, and often deploys it in combination with other chemicals. For example, Jessner's (a popular peel used in clinics) combines TCA with salicylic acid, lactic acid and resorcinol solution. Deep peels used to contain strong solvents like phenol, but these are rarely used these days, as patients need to be heavily sedated and recovery time can be months.

CRYOPEEL

Most people know about using liquid nitrogen to burn off warts and early skin cancers, but it is also possible to use super-cold liquid nitrogen (which has a temperature of around -196°C) on the skin's surface (called a cryopeel). As the skin temperature drops, any water in the skin turns to ice and blood stops flowing, akin to a frozen stream. This immediately triggers an inflammatory response, turning over not only the cold damage but any old skin as well, giving smoother, pinker, and tighter looking skin. The best results usually appear ten days or so after the procedure.

Skin cooling can be achieved using a spray gun or an implement something like a paintbrush. They apply the nitrogen in a spiral motion away from the centre of the area being treated. Sometimes a probe is cooled by a stream of nitrogen and then applied to the skin. The cosmetic results from freezing the skin's surface are said to be similar to that achieved by a chemical peel. In addition, by varying the exposure time, the pressure on the skin and/or the number and frequency of re-treatments, cryotherapy allows the practitioner to control how deep the (cryo)peel will go at any one point on the skin. This is like varying the strength and exposure time to a chemical peel. In this respect cryotherapy is more akin to dermabrasion. The super-cold nitrogen is only applied to the skin for a limited period of time, usually no more than thirty seconds and much less for areas with thinner skin. There is some pain during the freezing and afterwards when the blood rushes back to the skin to warm it, but this pain is usually short-lived and most treatments can be performed without any anaesthesia. For longer or more extensive treatments some clinicians prefer to use a local anaesthetic cream.

PRE-CONDITIONING FOR A PEEL

The right preparation is critical for getting the most out of a peel and reducing the risk of complications. Prepare the skin be using an AHA serum to create the perfect surface for all peels. It also helps to prevent hyperpigmentation forming. This is known as pre-conditioning or priming, and usually takes two to three weeks before the treatment, sometimes longer for those with a darker complexion. Priming will usually involve:

> Providing broad-spectrum sun protection from UV rays to protect the skin from sun damage.
> A daily skincare regimen to cleanse the skin.
> Application of moisturiser twice a day.
> Avoidance of artificial tanning agents, sun exposure and cigarette smoke.

Your practitioner may also recommend that you pre-treat the skin with retinoids, AHAs or vitamin C to help speed up the healing process after the procedure. Some practitioners recommend the use of topical steroids two to three days before certain peels and for up to two weeks after the treatment, to reduce the risk of swelling, depigmentation and bruising, especially with deep peels. To reduce the risk of blotchy pigmentation, practitioners may recommend the use of what are known as 'tyrosinase inhibitors'. These reduce the over production of the enzymes that are responsible for hyperpigmentation. They are typically started about two weeks before the peel and continued for two to three months after the peel. Hydroquinone and kojic acid may be prescribed; however, these ingredients do have side effects, so alternatives like oxyresveratrol are preferred. If you are prone to cold sores, then it is essential that you take your antiviral medication. Any time that the surface of the skin is disrupted a cold sore may erupt.

DURING AND AFTER THE PROCEDURE

SUPERFICIAL PEEL

Immediately prior to a superficial peel, the skin needs to be thoroughly cleansed and degreased (usually with alcohol or acetone) to remove makeup, moisturisers or facial oils that may interfere with the even penetration of the peeling agent. Your hair will also be covered, and goggles or eye patches are used to protect your eyes during the treatment. It is especially important that tears do not mix with and so dilute the acid in the peel, or wash the peel onto unprotected areas like the neck. Some practitioners use a thick layer of barrier gel to protect the neck, just in case. These steps are also required for deep and medium peels. Superficial peels do not require the use of anaesthesia or oral sedatives.

During the procedure, one or more chemical solutions are applied to the target area, using a disposable gauze square or cotton-tipped applicator. A superficial peel stays on the skin for anywhere from a few minutes to 20 minutes. The longer times are typically for those who have had the treatment before. (Medium and deep peels are left on the skin for longer periods of time.) When an adequate response has been achieved, the solution is neutralised and wiped off.

Most people can go back to their normal activities immediately after having a superficial peel. Superficial peels cause only mild discomfort and may involve slight redness, which fades quickly in a few hours. By the end of the first day after the treatment the skin may temporarily take on a light brown (tanned) appearance. By day three, peeling of the skin begins, which lasts for three to seven days (longer for non-facial peels). However, note that peeling does not always occur with superficial peels, but this doesn't mean it hasn't achieved results.

The deeper the peel the longer it may take for the skin to heal. It is important to note that the general health of the patient and their stress levels effect the rate at which the skin heals. Throughout the healing period it is advised that you use a good moisturiser (biomimetic), to ensure the appropriate repair of the skin, along with a broad-spectrum sunscreen. Makeup can be used during this period.

MEDIUM PEEL

A medium peel is also an outpatient procedure and is performed by a more experienced practitioner than is required for a superficial peel. Downtime for recovery is longer and there are more potential risks. Following the procedure, it is essential to use moisturiser as required in order to keep the skin moist and well-nourished during the peeling phase. The use of a broad-spectrum sunscreen is also essential. Results are always enhanced with the use of active cosmeceutical products containing AHAs, retinol and tyrosinase inhibitors during the recovery period.

DEEP PEEL

Deep peels do effectively burn the skin to trigger its regeneration. However, the skin will remain red for some weeks after the procedure. Deep peels must be performed by a doctor and are painful so typically an anaesthetic is required during the procedure and painkillers afterwards. Fans and cool compresses may also be used during the procedure to lessen the burning sensation caused by the chemicals. Deep peels are sometimes performed under a general anaesthetic.

There is also a risk of damage to the melanocyte cells (pigment forming cells) that can result in blotchy pigmentation. These risks, and the disruption to lifestyle that several months of healing can make, mean deep peels are rarely performed today.

Following treatment, a thick ointment will be applied to the skin, and sometimes bandages. A steroid-containing cream may be prescribed to reduce inflammation. Avoid excessive exposure to the sun until the peeling has stopped and use sunscreen with an SPF of at least 30 every day to avoid sun damage. Do not scrub or pick at the peeling skin. Premature peeling can increase the risk of complications and reduce the effectiveness of the treatment.

Realistic expectations need to be clear and, as with all treatments, a full consultation with an expert practitioner must be undertaken prior to treatment.

WHAT ARE THE POTENTIAL SIDE EFFECTS?

'Sex and the City' gave chemical peels a bad name. One horrified look at the raw, red and unattractive state of Samantha's skin as she leaves the clinic after what her doctor explains as a 'refreshing' chemical peel is enough to put women off the procedure for good. While it is true that many women will experience redness or swelling after a chemical peel, it is seldom severe or incapacitating unless a deep peel is performed poorly.

Whenever a procedure is performed there are risks involved. But providing all pre- and post-treatment care is followed, side effects are rare.

However, smokers are at risk of complications following these treatments as smoking lowers the capacity of the skin to heal itself. Those with medical conditions or who are taking medication that may make them more sensitive to the effects of the peel, may also need to avoid having a peel, or avoid certain peeling agents. Those using retinoids should cease their use 48 hours prior to the treatment and for between five and seven days afterwards in order to avoid additional skin sensitivity.

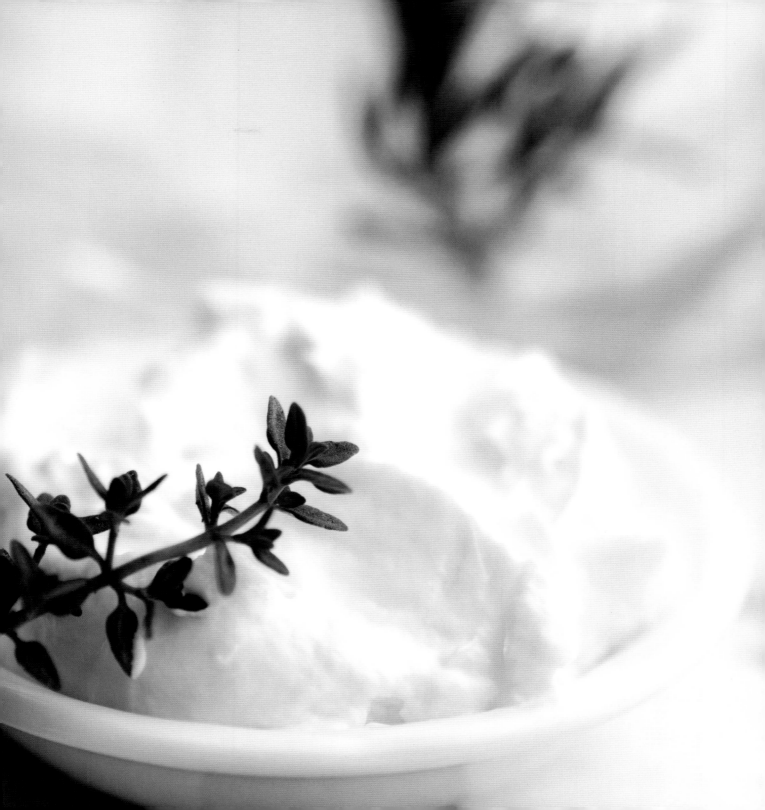

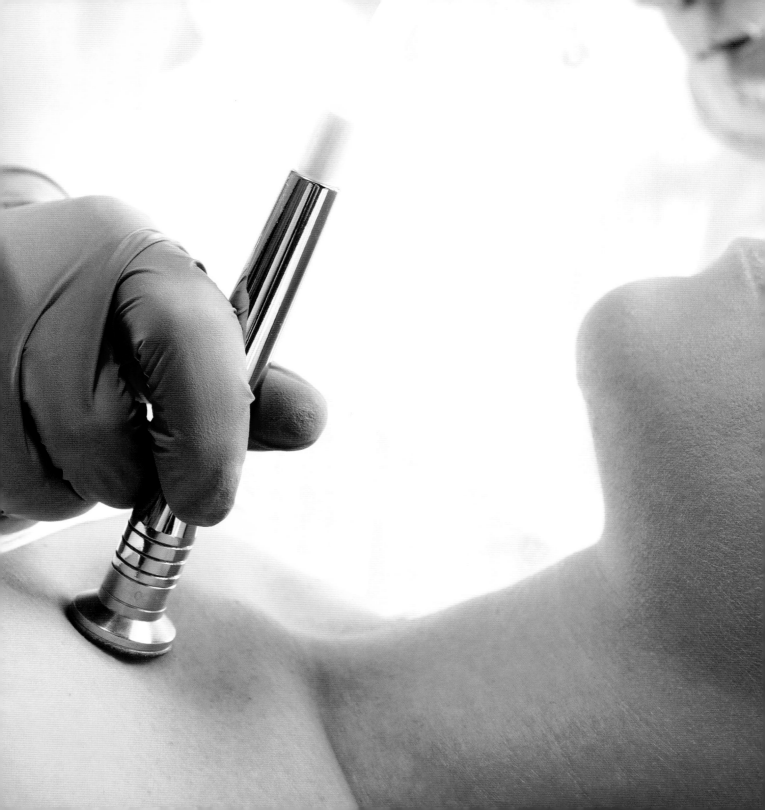

CHAPTER 26:

MICRODERMABRASION

Microdermabrasion is one of the most popular and straightforward resurfacing techniques. It involves rubbing off dead skin cells from the outer layer of the skin using abrasive substances, such as crystals, brushes or various sharp instruments. Dermabrasion is a very old technique. Even the ancient Egyptians used sandpaper to treat unsightly scars.

Microdermabrasion (or 'microderm' for short) is a modern invention that simply means selectively rubbing off only the outer dead layer of the skin's epidermis, similar to the effects of a superficial peel. The term dermabrasion today generally refers to aggressive abrading of the top and mid layers of our skin, akin to a deep peel for treating deep scars. This is generally a surgical procedure requiring an anaesthetic and prolonged recovery time. By contrast, microdermabrasion is far gentler (some say it feels like a cat licking your skin) and recovery time is very short.

MICRODERMABRASION PROCEDURE

Microdermabrasion is usually performed by spraying a stream of abrasive crystals onto the skin surface then almost immediately removing them with a vacuum. A number of different crystals are available. The most common are aluminium oxide, although salt crystals (sodium chloride), magnesium oxide, sodium bicarbonate, and organic grains made from plants are also used. Microdermabrasion can also be provided by hollow stainless wands with a diamond tip. This method does not spray crystals over the skin.

Typically, a professional microdermabrasion system consists of a high-pressure pump, a tube, a handpiece and a vacuum-like device. The handpiece that sprays the crystals or the hollow diamond tipped wand are applied to and moved over the skin. The vacuum device concurrently removes the exfoliated skin and also the crystals (in the case of crystal microdermabrasion). Some practitioners prefer to use only the vacuum-like tool to remove dead skin, without any crystals being deployed, in order to stimulate the skin and improve circulation; however, this is not technically microdermabrasion. Some machines use rotary brushes, scrubbing pads or a sonicating motion, similar that of electric toothbrushes, to do the same job.

Microdermabrasion's cosmetic effect is achieved partly by physically removing the outer dead cells (called exfoliation). This stimulates skin turnover, as with a peel. New, younger looking skin cells appear and work their way the surface, making the skin look and feel softer, smoother and healthier. By removing the old cells on the surface, microdermabrasion achieves a polishing or 'gloss' effect on the skin, as the dead skin cells are dry and non-reflective. This is why dermabrasion is particularly useful for women who have dull skin (a common characteristic of older skin). Some superficial skin imperfections such as fine lines, blotchiness, acne and blemishes can be improved with repeated microdermabrasion procedures. However, just like a superficial peel, microdermabrasion is not effective in the treatment of deep wrinkles, which involve changes to deeper skin layers and so require different interventions.

Unlike a peel, shearing the skin's surface with microdermabrasion also triggers the underlying skin to be more active in remodelling and repair. One study found that microdermabrasion, although it is classed as a superficial procedure, resulted in increased levels of growth factors in the deeper dermal layer of the skin. Finally, removing the outer layer of the skin can improve penetration of cosmeceuticals, enhancing their benefits.

As with all forms of resurfacing, the depth to which our skin is treated must be very precisely controlled. This is achieved by carefully adjusting the force of crystal flow, the rate of suction through the hollow stainless steel diamond wand, the speed of handpiece movement, and the number of passes over any part of the skin being treated. As in all areas of cosmetic medicine, it takes experience to get the optimal outcomes and minimise potential side effects.

Home microdermabrasion treatments use much the same kind of crystals as in professional treatments, but deliver them in creams and scrubs rather than in specialised mechanical devices. Consequently, the effects of home treatments are generally more modest than those achieved by professional procedures.

PREPARATION AND AFTERCARE FOR MICRODERMABRASION

Preparation for a microdermabrasion is minimal. For the week prior to the procedure, you should avoid excessive exposure to the sun and use a moisturising sun block with an SPF of at least 30. It is also advisable to stop taking warfarin, aspirin or anti-inflammatory drugs like NSAIDS (e.g. ibuprofen, ketoprofen) one to two weeks before the procedure in order to reduce the risk of bruising. Some practitioners also recommend stopping vitamin E, ginseng, fish-oil tablets and herbal supplements with anticoagulant effects for the same reason. A practitioner may also prefer their patients to stop taking oral contraceptives prior to the procedure, because of its effects on bleeding and clotting. If you have a history of herpes infection (cold sores) near the target area, you may be asked by the practitioner to take antiviral medication before the treatment. Anyone with an active herpes infection adjacent to the treatment area should delay the procedure.

Prior to each treatment the area of skin that will be targeted needs to be thoroughly cleansed to remove makeup, moisturiser, lotions, and oils.

Professional microdermabrasion procedures are usually done in a skin clinic, medical spa, or in the practitioner's office. The procedure itself is straightforward and generally painless. You may feel a little bit of tension from the abrasion and vacuuming. Topical anaesthesia or painkillers are generally not needed, but if required, numbing cream can be placed on the target area, left to penetrate for ten to 30 minutes, and then wiped off before the treatment is performed.

Because sharp crystals are flying around, everyone needs to wear protective eyewear. It is also important not to inhale the crystals.

During the treatment, the practitioner will press the microdermabrasion tool against your skin. This hand device will smoothly pass over your skin around two to four times, over the course of ten to 40 minutes, depending on the size of the area being treated, and the desired depth of treatment.

There's no downtime for recovery required after a microdermabrasion procedure, so it is possible to go back to your normal activities immediately. Your skin may be slightly pinkish straight after the procedure, but this usually subsides after a few hours. If you feel uncomfortable, you can apply a cold compress or an ice pack to the treated area to help reduce the pain. Persistent redness after the procedure is responsive to weak steroid creams.

As with a peel, it is important to protect the treated skin from excessive sunlight, because the new skin cells that emerge during the healing process are prone to sun damage for a few weeks while the skin is recovering and remodelling. It is common to use specialised lotions, creams and moisturisers to hydrate the skin between treatment sessions, but use only skincare products that are approved by your practitioner.

The 'gloss' effect of microdermabrasion may be noticeable right after your first treatment session. The skin should also appear healthier, smoother and softer. However, these effects are only temporary. Your skin renews around every 30 days, microdermabrasion is usually repeated every two to four weeks.

POTENTIAL SIDE EFFECTS OF MICRODERMABRASION

Microdermabrasion has few side effects, and any that do occur are minor and usually subside within 24 hours after the treatment. These can include redness, itching and a mild sunburn-like sensation. Flaking of the skin may appear after two to four days. After the treatment, your skin will be more sensitive to the sun. Most side effects result from the healing skin undergoing excessive sun exposure, leading to redness, itching and dryness. These effects can be avoided by staying out of strong sunlight and applying appropriate sunscreen and moisturiser. If you have used Roaccutane® or other drugs that increase the skin's sensitivity to light (such as amiodarone or allopurinol) within the past six months, then you should not undergo microdermabrasion.

Another side effect of microdermabrasion can be the increased appearance of acne. This is a natural reaction to microdermabrasion since the pores are unclogged during the treatment and this releases acne-causing bacteria; however, it is short-lived if it occurs at all.

Overzealous or inexperienced use of microdermabrasion can in rare cases lead to bruising, scarring or the appearance of dark or light patches on the skin, especially in Asian or dark-skinned women. Always go to a well-trained, experienced practitioner.

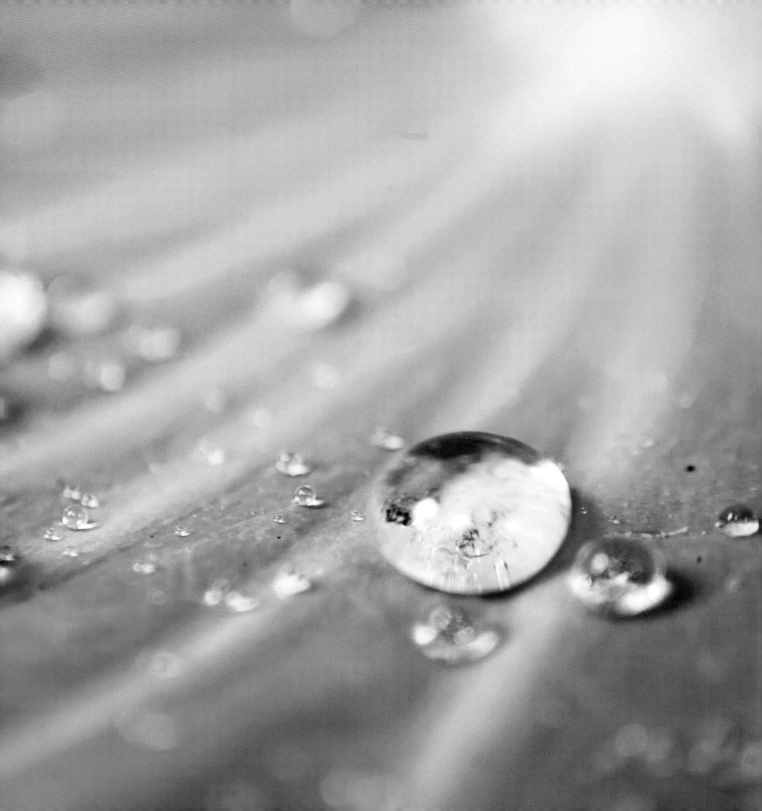

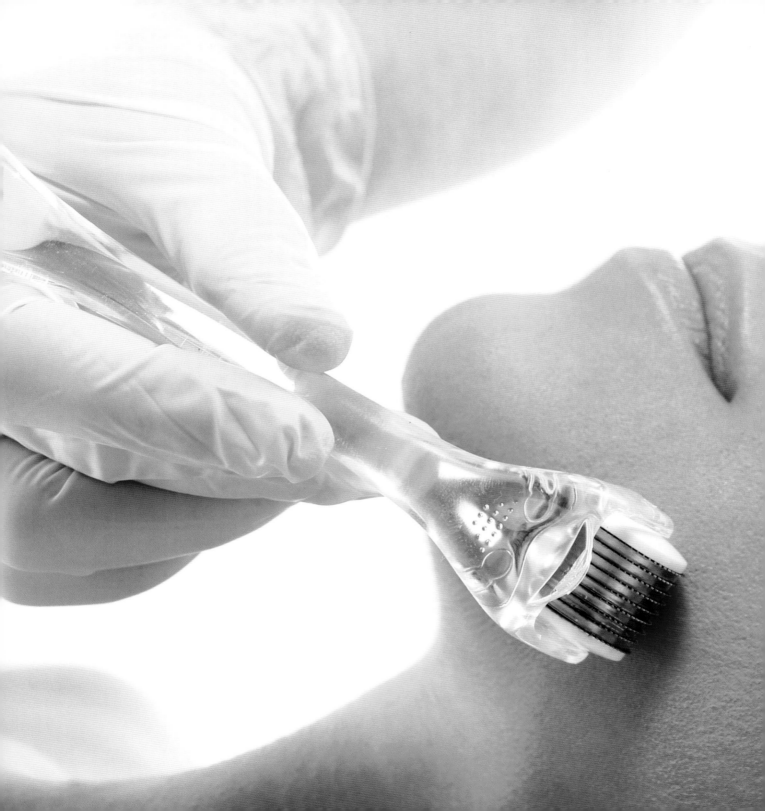

CHAPTER 27

MICRONEEDLING

Getting beneficial chemicals into the skin is not easy. Conventional (hypodermic) needles work, but they are painful when pricked into and under the skin. Another approach is to create very tiny holes through the outer layers of the skin with miniature microneedles, which enables beneficial chemicals to be delivered to where they will have the greatest effect.

There are different kinds of microneedles used in cosmetic medicine. Each is very tiny, about the same width as an acupuncture needle. Their length depends on the type of skin being treated and the area being targeted. For example, thinner, more fragile skin will generally receive needles 0.5 millimetres long, while for the treatment of scarring needles of between two and three millimetres may be deployed to reach the deeper dermis.

Unlike conventional needles, the microneedles used in cosmetic medicine are solid (with no hole in the middle) and formed into sheets of needles which are applied as a stamp (e.g. Dermastamp™) or using a roller (such as Dermaroller or MTSRoller™). Some reusable rollers are available for home use. There are also microneedling pens that can be used to deploy the needles.

Each needle punctures a small hole in the outer layer of the skin that stays open for about a day before fully closing. These provide temporary conduits (known as microchannels) enabling topical agents to penetrate into lower layers of the skin. Sometimes the needles are coated with an agent, which is delivered into the skin when the needle is applied.

It has also been demonstrated that micro-injuries caused by microneedling can stimulate matrix formation in the deeper layers of the skin, even without using any chemicals or topical agents. In fact, microneedling is sometimes marketed as collagen induction therapy (CIT), serving as a kind of volumiser by promoting collagen production to improve the elasticity, firmness and tone of the skin, as well as reduce lines and wrinkles. Microneedling is also used to treat scarring, like acne scarring, stretchmarks or a scar formed after a deep wound.

MICRONEEDLING PROCEDURE

Preparation for microneedling is minimal. Stopping warfarin, aspirin or anti-inflammatory drugs, like NSAIDS (e.g. ibuprofen, ketoprofen) one to two weeks before the procedure will reduce the risk of bruising. Some practitioners also recommend stopping vitamin E, ginseng, fish-oil tablets, and herbal supplements with anticoagulant effects for the same reason. Prior to each treatment the area of skin to be targeted needs to be thoroughly cleansed to remove makeup or any other material that may interfere with the effectiveness of the treatment.

When using CIT, it is common to use topical local anaesthetic or a cold compress beforehand to numb the area. However, because the tiny microneedles don't penetrate particularly deeply, the procedure is minimally uncomfortable, mainly in bony areas such as the forehead.

The practitioner will make a series of injections, usually utilising a roller or stamp coated with thousands of microneedles, each of which is only a few millimetres long.

There's little or no downtime for recovery after microneedling and it is possible to quickly return to your normal activities. Patients are advised to avoid anything that creates heat in the skin, including intensive exercise or hot showers or baths for 24 hours afterwards. It is also advised that patients do not touch their treated skin for one hour after the procedure and don't apply makeup for at least six hours. Most clinics will recommend the use of a specialised post-needling kit (typically containing a cleanser, serums and chemical-free sun protection) for at least three to five days following the procedure, after which patients can go back to their regular skincare regimen.

A course of three treatments is typically recommended and they are usually performed six to eight weeks apart. A top-up treatment every six to twelve months helps to maintain results. When treating scarring it may take up to five treatments to reach the desired result.

SIDE EFFECTS OF MICRONEEDLING

After microneedling it is common to experience temporary swelling and redness, a little like mild sunburn; this usually settles within 12 to 24 hours. Small bruises may also occur if deep needles injure superficial capillaries. Some patients may experience dehydration and mild flaking of the skin in the days after the treatment. This can be reduced with the application of hyaluronic acid and moisturising creams. Holes in the skin theoretically make it possible for bacteria to get in and cause infections, although this is generally unlikely unless the treated area is already compromised. Because there is no heating of the skin, there is less risk of post-inflammatory pigmentation (which can occur with laser treatment) and so all skin types can be treated with microneedling. To reduce the risks and to get the best results, always look for practitioners who have undergone specialised skin needling training.

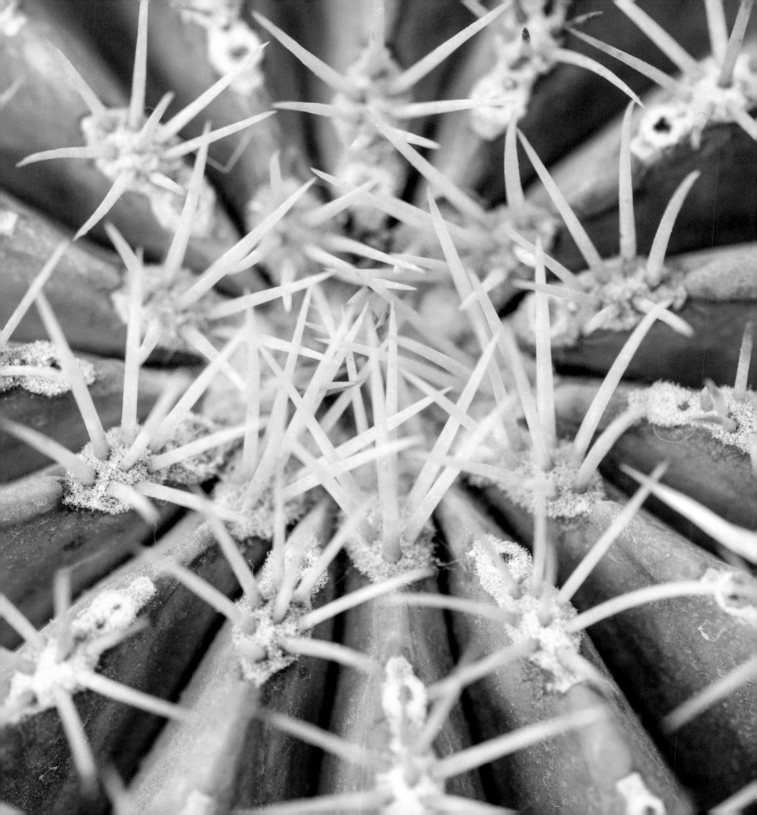

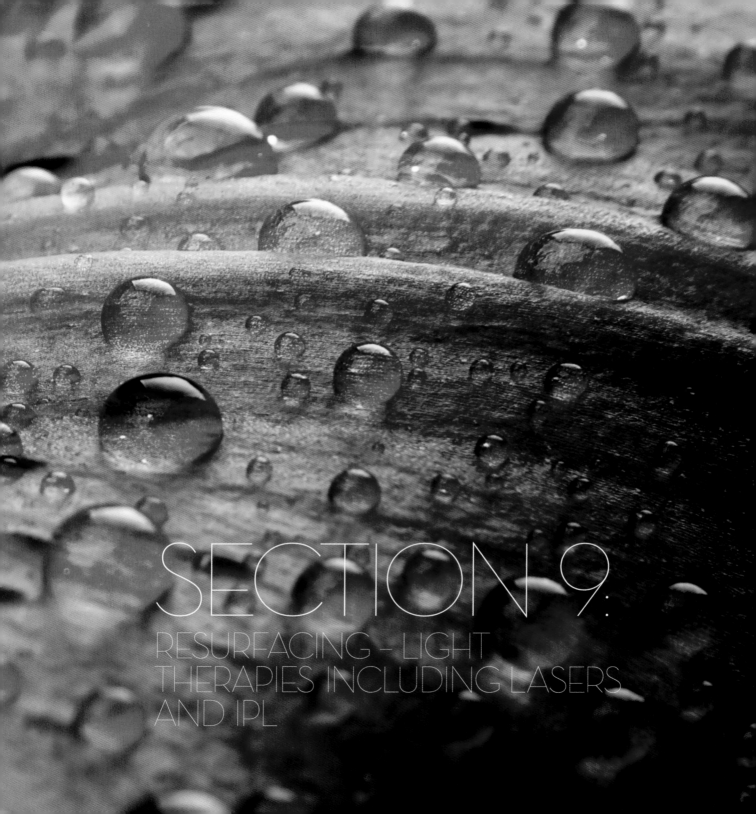

SECTION 9:

RESURFACING – LIGHT THERAPIES INCLUDING LASERS AND IPL

CHAPTER 28: LED THERAPIES
CHAPTER 29: LASER RESURFACING
CHAPTER 30: INTENSE PULSED LIGHT (IPL)

Light therapies can be divided into two overall categories: laser therapies and intense pulsed light (IPL) therapies. Lasers are more specific in their actions than IPL, but both are useful in rejuvenating skin and can be used for hair removal. Generally speaking, all light therapies rely on the process of photothermolysis. This works on the principle that light of a particular wavelength will be attracted to a particular chromophore or colour. Think of wearing a black T-shirt on the beach (the chromophore) and how the sunlight (light wavelength) is attracted to the black colour, meaning that the shirt heats up more than a white one, from which the light is reflected rather than absorbed.

When you heat up a chromophore in the skin, you disrupt it and tissue damage occurs. The chromophores are generally referred to as the 'target', and when treating skin the targets are usually melanin (cause of pigmentation disorders such as sun damage and melasma), haemoglobin (which creates vascular presentations such as port wine stain, rosacea and facial and leg capillaries) and water (wrinkles and scars).

They key to successful laser and IPL treatment is the expertise of the operator, not in the type of machine used. This is because a well-trained and experienced clinician will understand what your skin issues are, what your current and past health history is, your Fitzpatrick Skin Type, the capabilities and safety considerations of the machines they use and how to adjust the therapeutic parameters on them to get the best result for you. The therapeutic parameters are the wavelength(s) required, the amount of energy needed, how to deliver the energy into the skin and what spot size is needed to reach the required depth. How your skin is treated will vary from treatment to treatment and requires a discerning clinician who has good critical thinking skills. There is no one machine, one setting or one way to treat a skin condition with lasers and IPL.

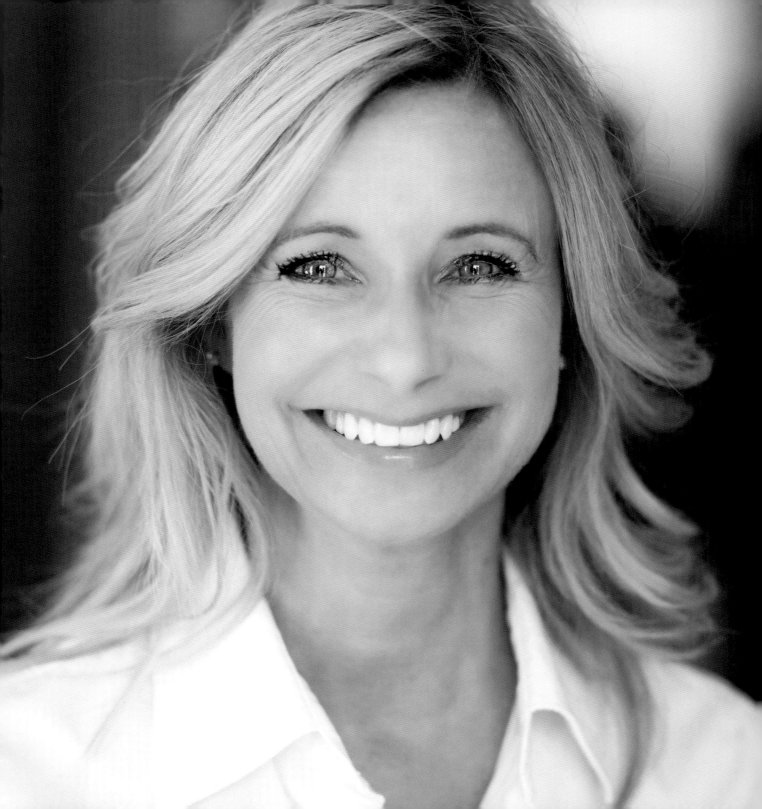

CHAPTER 28

LED THERAPIES

There are many different ways to apply concentrated light onto our skin. We don't always have to use lasers. One of the most popular methods in recent years has to been to use light emitting diodes (LEDs). The technology actually originated at NASA, but since around the year 2000 it has been deployed to treat photoaged skin.

LED therapy involves aiming concentrated light of specific wavelengths onto the skin. This is sometimes known as low-level light therapy. Unlike a conventional laser therapy that is designed to heat or burn holes, low-level light therapy uses wavelengths of light that do not cause damage to the skin, but rather promote healing. Compared to laser treatments, this allows much larger areas of skin to be treated equally, smoothly and gently.

HOW DOES LED THERAPY WORK?

Most cosmetic phototherapy devices using LEDs work by directing light that is at the red and infrared waveband of the spectrum onto the skin. We see the light in the visible range of this part of the spectrum as red. The other part is beyond the limits of our vision, and is referred to as near-infrared light. These parts of the spectrum are able to penetrate deeply into the skin (with the infrared going deeper than the red). It has the benefit of triggering changes in the way the skin functions (known as photobiomodulation) without heating or otherwise damaging the skin. One reason that this might be the case is that the LED tricks the skin into thinking it has been getting some extra sunlight in that beneficial waveband. However, in LED therapy there is no ultraviolet (UV) light, which is the part of the spectrum of sunlight that can cause skin damage, inflammation, pigmentation and even cancer with excessive exposure. So LED therapy is really just like getting outdoors in the sunshine while wearing a really high factor sun cream, offering concentrated benefits, but without the risks.

Three things happen to photobiomodulated cells: if they are damaged or compromised, like in ageing skin, then they will be repaired; if a cell has a job to do, like the cells that manufacture collagen, then they will do it better and faster; finally, if there are not enough cells for a particular purpose, then more will be called in to the area. Any one, or all three of these beneficial events can happen in LED therapy.

This means that it is an effective treatment for rejuvenating skin which is showing the signs of ageing – by, for instance, reducing wrinkles, correcting sun damage and pigmentation, and reducing the appearance of redness, visible capillaries and blemishes. It can also be used to treat some forms of scarring, acne, stretch marks, psoriasis and dermatitis.

WHAT TO EXPECT FROM LED THERAPY TREATMENT

The procedure itself is very simple. You sit under a panel of LEDs of the right wavelength (or colour) for between five and 20 minutes. Depending on the skin condition being treated, an initial course of LED therapy is usually performed twice a week over four weeks. 'Top up' sessions can then be administered every few weeks to retain and enhance the skin rejuvenation process.

LED therapy can be administered by a clinician or a beauty therapist. Often, beauty therapists will have a tanning bed or similar equipment that can be utilised for administering LED therapy (and LED has not been linked to melanoma, as tanning beds in the past have been). Some people find the whole procedure quite calming, like lying out in the sun (only without the nasty UV!). Indeed, patients have even been known to fall asleep while undergoing the therapy.

LED therapy is suitable for all skin types and the level of light used is insufficient to cause pigmentation or loss of pigmentation. This makes it safe for patients of any age, not only those wishing to combat the signs of ageing, but also younger patients who require treatment for acne or scarring. While not the cheapest of cosmetic skin treatments, LED therapy is a fairly affordable option for those looking for a non-invasive method of skin rejuvenation.

No particular preparation is needed for an LED therapy session except that the area being treated needs to be well cleaned. The clinician or therapist administering the treatment will typically use a cleaning agent before applying the light. Some practitioners also recommend that antioxidants (topical or oral) be stopped for a few weeks prior to the procedure to maximise its effects. It is not necessary to stop anti-inflammatories or blood thinners, provided they contain no component that might cause photosensitivity in the skin, which applies particularly to the visible red spectrum. The same is true for certain prescription or over-the-counter medications. Many medications – and cosmetics such as anti-ageing creams – can cause photosensitivity in the skin which, when exposed to red LED light (rather than near-infrared LEDs), can make the skin more prone to damage. As such, if you are taking any medications, talk to your GP before starting LED therapy.

ARE THERE ANY SIDE EFFECTS?

There are no significant side effects associated with LED therapy. Because there is no skin damage involved with the treatment, bleeding and bruising are not a problem.

While there is no specific recovery time required with LED therapy, it is advisable to stay out of direct sunlight for a few hours after the treatment.

Avoid any treatments that claim to offer other parts of the light spectrum in combination with red. Some systems add blue, green or yellow light, but these wavelengths simply don't penetrate deeply enough into the skin to have any beneficial effect in terms of rejuvenation of the deeper dermal skin cells (although yellow light does have some benefits for certain cells in the epidermis). They may be useful as a secondary treatment before or after the LED therapy, but in general should not be applied at the same time. This can confuse the skin cells and limit the effectiveness of the treatment.

ARE THERE ANY LIMITATIONS?

LED therapy is very simple and cheap, with no pain or recovery downtime, and is safe for all skin types. However, it is sometimes considered – somewhat unjustifiably – as an alternative therapy when compared to things like laser, ultrasound and radiofrequency.

It is true that, compared to these other treatments, LED therapy does not have the same immediate impact in terms of skin rejuvenation – it requires time, with several sessions over several weeks, and often the best results of the treatment developing incrementally up to 12 weeks and beyond the final treatment in the series.

However, clinical trials have confirmed that LED therapy is effective in reducing wrinkles, smoothing the appearance of the skin, and combatting other cosmetic signs of ageing.

Clinical studies have also shown that LED therapy is often most effective when used in combination with other rejuvenating skin treatments. It has been used in conjunction with surgical procedures to enhance wound healing and reduce inflammation and swelling. However, the effectiveness of LED therapy can also be improved when used in concert with other cosmetic skin treatments, such as facial peels, microdermabrasion, and good quality complementary skincare cosmeceuticals.

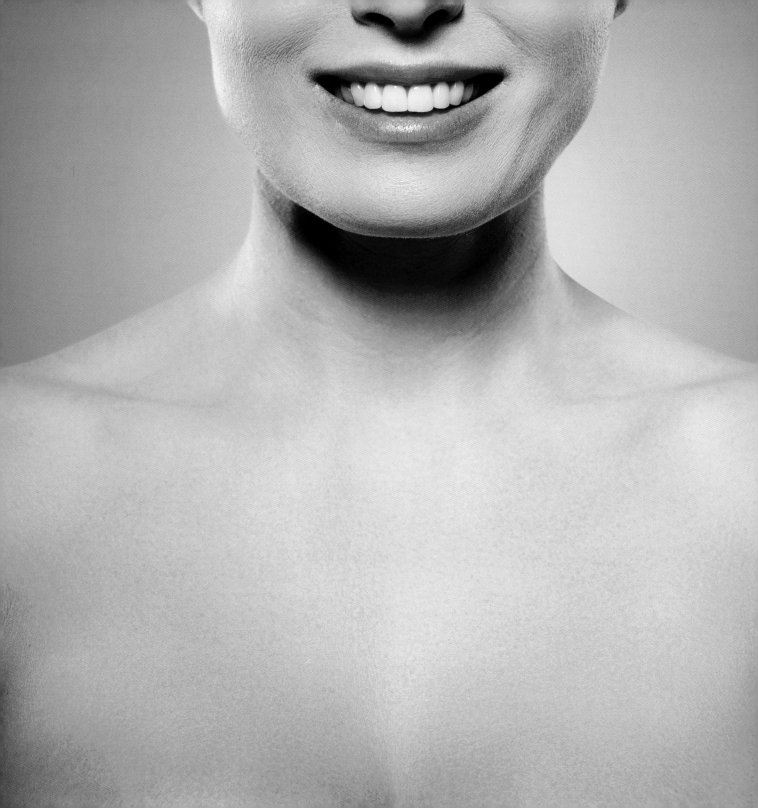

CHAPTER 29

LASER RESURFACING

Laser has become one of the most widely used modalities to treat ageing skin. It works by directing a high-energy beam of light at a particular skin area to selectively heat and disrupt skin cells, while leaving other areas of the skin unaffected (this is technically known as selective photothermolysis). This precision allows it to be used in many different ways and to target many different parts of the skin.

ABLATIVE LASER THERAPY

One of the uses of lasers is to literally vaporise the outer surface of the skin to a very precise depth. This is commonly known as a laser peel or ablative laser therapy. The principle is the same as for other resurfacing techniques like chemical peels and dermabrasion – to remove the skin cells from the surface. Only here there are no chemicals and no abrasives, just laser beams.

The most commonly used ablative lasers are the Carbon Dioxide laser (CO_2) and the Erbium:YAG laser. The CO_2 laser is the preferred treatment for deep wrinkles, scars and birthmarks. The Erbium:YAG laser removes mild to moderate wrinkles and lines on the face as well as on the neck, chest and hands.

One advantage of ablative laser treatment is that while the outer layers of the epidermis are destroyed, a lot of heat is generated in the skin. This heat affects the dermis, causing the collagen matrix to contract. This tightens the skin, which is why laser resurfacing is often also known as a non-surgical facelift (although its effects are more modest than its surgical counterpart). The wounding process stimulates an inflammatory response that removes the old damaged collagen and replaces it with new healthy matrix, which is more organised and flexible, which means increased elasticity and strength and an improved smoother, tighter appearance.

The problem with ablative lasers is that vaporising the outer part of the skin and creating a wound can be associated with significant side effects including pain, redness, swelling, pigmentation, scarring and possible infection. It also can require an anaesthetic and significant downtime for recovery in some cases (see below), although the end results are very satisfactory for most women. Nevertheless, the popularity of ablative laser appears to be on the decline as more women seek out safer procedures that require less downtime.

NON-ABLATIVE LASER THERAPY

An alternative approach for resurfacing, although much less effective, is the use of non-ablative lasers. This heats the deeper layers in the skin while at the same time cooling the outer (epidermis) surface (with a gel, cold handpiece or spray cooling devices) so that it doesn't get damaged. This means that you don't get a wound or a scar, and it significantly reduces the chance of infection and other side effects that occur when using ablative treatments. At the same time, selective injury to the deeper layers of the skin still triggers increased production of collagen and other matrix proteins to regenerate the skin. Contraction of the matrix in response to heating also results in some skin tightening, but it is not a facelift. If tightening is what you need then it is best combined with anti-wrinkle injections and/or fillers. Lasers do not melt fillers, and may in fact enhance their longevity. On its own, the ultimate effect on appearance of non-ablative laser therapy is generally less pronounced than that achieved with ablative techniques, especially for deep wrinkles around the eyes and mouth. Multiple treatments (usually three to five) may be required to produce the desired results, but this procedure does have the advantage of fewer complications and less downtime for recovery.

FRACTIONAL LASER THERAPY

Rather than vaporising a whole area of skin, as with the ablative CO_2 and erbium lasers mentioned above, another approach treats only a fraction of the skin (around 20 percent) by making a number of microscopic wounds with a laser. This is known as fractional laser therapy. Unlike with non-ablative lasers, there are holes in the skin, but because of the tiny size of the holes, the fact that they are tapered (bigger on the inside than the outside), and the retention of healthy skin adjacent to the treated area, any wounds heal very quickly and will recover within one or two days following the procedure. Healing is usually complete within a week. This means fewer and shorter side effects than an ablative laser treatment, less downtime for recovery and minimal post-treatment care. In expert hands, the results are often better, quicker and more sustained than those achieved with a standard non-ablative laser. Also fewer re-treatments are typically required, which has meant that fractional laser therapy has become extremely popular over recent years. Blended treatments that combine non-ablative lasers with fractional lasers in a few key spots are also popular.

PHOTODYNAMIC THERAPY (PDT)

Another way of harnessing the selective targeting power of lasers and other light sources is photodynamic therapy. In this procedure a chemical is applied to the skin to increase its sensitivity to light and to cause the selected cells to be disrupted and die. This means that much less light needs to be applied to get the desired effect, and other (healthy) areas get so little light they are unaffected. It is mostly used for treating skin cancers and pre-cancerous lesions such as actinic keratoses, although it can be used to selectively target and remove ugly skin pores or hair.

PREPARATION FOR LASER THERAPY

Preparation for laser treatment is minimal but important. For the fortnight prior to the procedure, you should avoid excessive exposure to the sun and regularly use a moisturising sun block with an SPF of at least 30. It is also recommended that you avoid artificial tanning agents and exfoliating agents for at least a week prior to undergoing laser treatment. Some clinics may recommend that you cease topical retinoids and vitamin A products too. If you take oral retinoids such as Roaccutane® you will have to cease taking them six months prior to laser treatment.

For pigmented areas, it is often recommended that topical bleaching agents (like hydroquinone), or preparations with pigment reducing antioxidants such as vitamin C and E are applied to the area being treated for at least a fortnight prior to the procedure, then resumed once the skin has healed and continued for at least six months. This can help reduce the risk of excessive pigmentation as a side effect.

Some practitioners also perform a skin analysis using imaging technology prior to the procedure, to help them choose the right laser, wavelengths and the treatment settings for your needs. Taking a photo beforehand is also important, so you see what you looked like (not just remember it) and assess the improvement. This is the best way to appreciate what a procedure can offer for you, and help you decide if you want to do it again. If you are prone to cold sores, preventive antiviral medication may be recommended for you prior to and after treatment.

WHAT HAPPENS DURING THE PROCEDURE?

Prior to each laser procedure the area of skin to be targeted needs to be thoroughly cleansed to remove any makeup or any material that may interfere with the treatment. Throughout the treatment session, you will wear protective eyewear. Insertion of full metal eye shields over the eyeball may be required for some treatments undertaken around the eyes.

The laser device is then placed over the skin being targeted. This device releases precise and intense flashes, or pulses, of light to heat the skin and trigger the growth of new cells.

The requirement for an anaesthetic depends on the kind of laser treatment you are having (ablative, non-ablative or fractional) and the length of the procedure, which may be anywhere from 20 minutes to two hours, depending on the size of the target area. Some laser treatments do not require any analgesia. Analgesia used incorrectly can actually dull your pain senses and increase the chances of burning, scarring and pigmentation changes. For some laser treatments, a numbing cream (topical anaesthetic) is placed on the target area, is left to penetrate for up to 30 minutes, and then removed before the treatment is performed. The sensation of the laser is then reduced to manage your discomfort. The laser device may be applied over an area multiple times and increases in heat with each pass; at the same time a cooling device cools the surface of the skin to ensure you are comfortable.

Nerve blocks are sometimes required for ablative therapies or fractional laser on high settings (to treat deep wrinkles). This involves an injection of an anaesthetic agent adjacent to the nerve that runs back from the area being treated, so no pain signals can reach your brain. For full laser resurfacing more effective pain control may be necessary, with a general anaesthetic or heavy sedation requiring the presence of a medical officer.

RECOVERY AND AFTERCARE FOR LASER TREATMENT

ABLATIVE LASER THERAPY

This more aggressive therapy means more downtime for recovery and more involved post-procedure care in order to prevent complications – involving wound care, soaks and painkillers as required. A short course of broad-spectrum oral antibiotic, and occasionally anti-viral tablets, is taken to reduce the risk of infection. A couple of weeks off from your usual activities is often required. Redness and swelling may take a month or two to fully settle.

NON-ABLATIVE LASER

There's little or no downtime for recovery required after a non-ablative laser procedure and you can immediately return to your normal activities. Your skin may be slightly pink or mildly swollen after the treatment, but this usually subsides after a few hours. If you feel uncomfortable, you may apply a cold compress or an ice pack to the treated area to help reduce pain and swelling. The remains of the pigmented lesion are slowly exfoliated over a week or two. The shed skin can look like coffee grounds. To reduce the risk of scarring, do not pick these or try to rub them off. In addition, do not use hot water when you shower or bathe for at least two days after the treatment as your skin may be sensitive to temperature.

FRACTIONAL LASER

After a fractional laser procedure, it is common to feel and look sunburnt and swollen. The heat sensation lasts approximately two to four hours post-procedure and can be managed with cool towels and fans if needed. Redness and swelling tend to be worst one to two days after the procedure, but usually resolve themselves quickly and are almost always gone by the end of a week.

Immediately after the treatment there may be oozing, pinpoint bleeding and crusting. It is recommended that you keep the wound moisturised until it has healed. By day four, you should start to shed the vaporised skin. This shedding can last a day or two. (Please note that in the very rare instance that you attain a burn greater than 3 millimetres on the face or hands or a burn in other areas larger than a 50-cent coin (3 centimetres in diameter) you should seek professional medical attention.)

For all laser therapy, it is important to stay out of the sun during the recovery phase, especially within the first few days, which is critical time for healing. This is because the new skin cells that emerge during the healing process are more prone to sun damage, and stimulation of melanin cells by the sun may cause excessive, unwanted pigmentation.

WHAT SIDE EFFECTS CAN OCCUR WITH LASER TREATMENT?

This really depends on the kind of laser treatment undertaken and its intensity. Non-ablative and fractional lasers have few side effects, but they may include:

> Break out of cold sores (herpes simplex virus)
> Prolonged redness
> Hypo- or hyper-pigmentation
> Textural change
> Dragging of the skin under the eye due to contraction of the collagen fibres (known as an ectropion)
> Scar tissue e.g. hypertrophic, atopic or keloid

While ablative laser resurfacing is highly effective, the risks of these complications are significantly greater with this type of procedure. In addition, disruption of the protective surface layer of the skin creates the risk of bacterial, viral or fungal infections.

Laser can reactivate the herpes simplex virus. To reduce this risk, every client with a history of cold sores will usually be given antiviral medications prior to the procedure. If you have an active cold sore you will be advised not to have the treatment.

Immediately after a laser treatment it is common to experience side effects like heat, redness and swelling. With non-ablative or fractional procedures, this usually lasts no more than a week. However, redness may be stubbornly persistent following some ablative procedures, lasting several months in some unfortunate cases. Uncommon side effects include mild blistering (less than three millimetres in size), slight pinpoint bleeding or bruising.

Some patients may experience whitening of the skin (known as hypo-pigmentation), especially on very tanned individuals. Clinicians may perform a test spot to check if the procedure will cause any lightening of the skin. Other patients may experience an increase in the pigmentation of treated areas (known as hyper-pigmentation). This is more likely when treating the neck and chest rather than the face. However, any hyper-pigmentation is usually transient and the rejuvenating skin will typically return to its normal skin tone within two to three months. Hypo-pigmentation may never resolve. Protect the treated areas from excessive sunlight after laser treatment to reduce the risk of pigmentation.

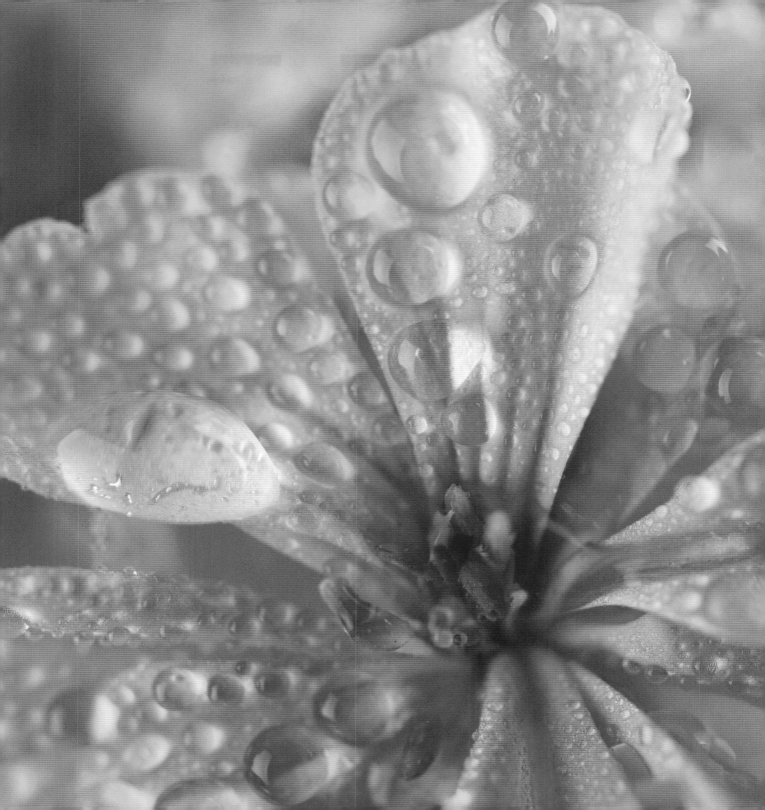

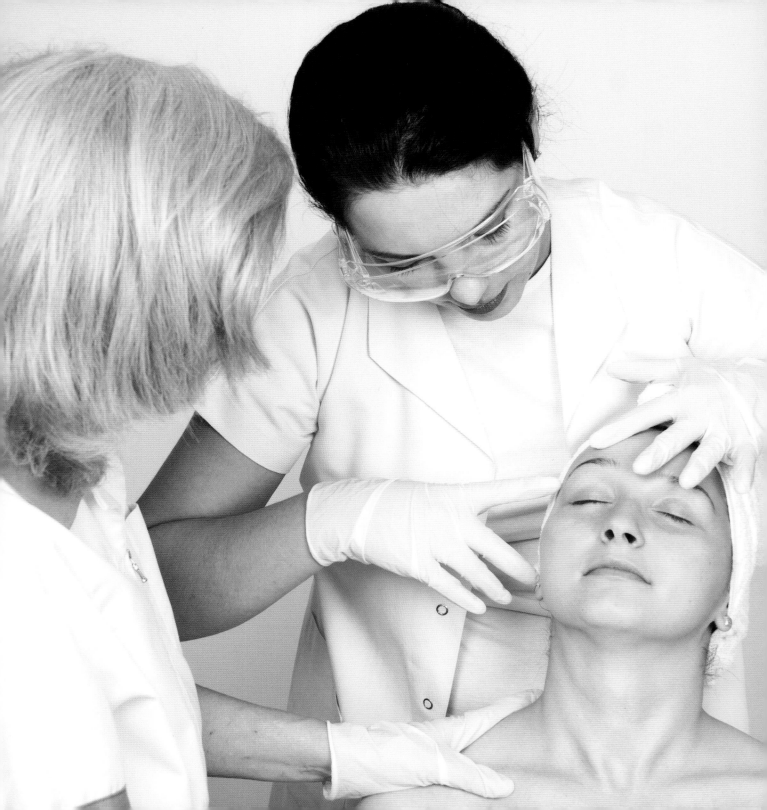

CHAPTER 30

INTENSE PULSED LIGHT (IPL)

Intense Pulsed Light (IPL) is another rejuvenation technique that is commonly used to improve the appearance of damaged and ageing skin. Instead of a laser, a high intensity beam of light is generated by passing an electrical current through a chamber filled with xenon gas. This light is then filtered and focused directly onto the skin. Certain elements in the skin are able to absorb these specific wavelengths of light, causing them to heat up, while other parts of the skin are less affected. This means that the photo-rejuvenation action can occur deep in the skin (in the dermis) while the outer surface is not disrupted (thus, IPL is classified as a non-ablative treatment).

IPL produces cosmetic effects similar to those of laser treatments; however, it is different from laser in how specifically it can target the chromophore of interest. Note, too, that IPL cannot resurface skin or remove tattoos.

Within each pulse, IPL flashes out light over a range of wavelengths (lasers deliver a burst of light at one specific wavelength). Laser light is more specific than the multiple wavelengths of IPL that bombard the skin; however, the same IPL device can be used to treat different targets by using 'cut-off filters'. These limit the wavelength reaching the skin to more selectively target the element in our skin that needs treating.

The same IPL device can be used to simultaneously treat different kinds of skin problems that would otherwise require different lasers. This versatility means that IPL is popular in many cosmetic medicine clinics (especially those not wanting to set up a range of different laser machines or to gain licensure to operate a Class 3B or 4 laser).

The other difference is the size of the area being treated with IPL. Lasers generally have smaller spot sizes to treat the skin. The IPL spot size (or footprint) is larger, so IPL treatments are generally faster than lasers, particularly when treating large areas. However, more IPL sessions are generally required to achieve the desired effect when compared to laser treatments.

The heat generated by IPL is also able to trigger the injury and remodelling of collagen in the dermis (known as denaturation). Wavelengths in the infrared spectrum are absorbed by water in the skin, which sets off inflammatory responses that remove old or damaged collagen and replace it with new healthy matrix, leading to at least partial replacement of the volume of the skin lost with age. This means a subtle, tighter, smoother texture, and increased softness with reduced lines. The effects on wrinkles are less dramatic than with injections of botulinum toxin or dermal fillers, and often require multiple treatment sessions to achieve the desired effect. Combining injectables and IPL and other light based treatments can be combined to good effect.

IPL can also be used to treat pigmented area (like age spots and sun spots) or unwanted blood vessels or redness on the face, legs or other parts of the body. Sometimes, practitioners use IPL as the light source for photodynamic therapy, in combination with methyl aminolevulenic acid (MAL), which acts to sensitise the skin to the effects of IPL. This is sometimes known as 'photodynamic photorejuvenation.'

WHAT TO EXPECT BEFORE AND DURING IPL

As with laser treatments, preparation is minimal but important, including avoiding excessive sunlight, artificial tanning agents and exfoliating agents for at least a week prior to the treatment.

IPL can occasionally stimulate a cold sore breakout if the herpes simplex virus affects you. A breakout can be avoided by taking an antiviral medication as a preventive measure before the procedure.

Some clinics will offer an anaesthetic cream to numb the area being treated 30 minutes or so prior to treatment. But be aware that anaesthetic use may numb your pain response and contribute to a burn, blister or scar. It is not advised to use anaesthetic when treating blood vessels as it may reduce how well a treatment works by causing constriction of blood vessels.

IPL generates heat in the skin, therefore the procedure also requires some form of cooling to be applied to the outer surface of the skin (the epidermis) to reduce the risk of damage and improve the efficiency of light delivery into the deeper dermis. This is usually done with a cooling gel or spray that is built into the handpiece that the practitioner uses to deliver the IPL.

Because there is heating (and cooling) occurring in the skin, it is common to feel some slight discomfort – a warm sensation that feels like someone is flicking you with an elastic band. Treatments last between three and ten minutes, and as soon as the treatment is finished, any discomfort quickly disappears with no residual effects.

The number of treatments and the interval between them will vary from person to person and problem to problem. On average, three to six treatments are required, performed every few weeks, and regular maintenance is recommended. The effect is cumulative for pigmented areas and generally continues until the treated area blends sufficiently into the surrounding skin. This will depend on the size and location of the area, how dark the area being treated is and the darkness of the surrounding skin.

Treated blood vessels will usually rapidly disappear, and the skin will look normal soon after the procedure. Occasionally, treated blood vessels may reappear in the days following a treatment. Multiple treatments may be required to completely destroy the vessel.

WHAT SIDE EFFECTS CAN OCCUR WITH IPL?

Recovery is rapid after the procedure, and it is possible to go back to your normal activities soon afterwards. Most IPL side effects are minor and subside within 24 hours. These include transient itching and redness, and mild swelling (especially with vascular treatments), which can persist for a few hours but is easily covered with makeup. There may also be some peeling of the skin for a few days after the treatment.

After the procedure, dark areas being treated may get a little darker instead of getting lighter. This is known as microcrusting. It is nothing to be worried about and is a sign that the treatment is working. It will settle after the old skin cells are pushed to the surface and peel off, which typically happens within seven to fourteen days, depending on the body area being treated. This process may be accelerated by applying a moisturiser twice a day or by performing micro-dermabrasion of the treated area one to two days following the procedure. Some patients may also experience pigment changes, with the treated area becoming lighter or darker. This is less common when therapeutic parameters such as the wavelength, energy and pulse duration are carefully titrated to your Fitzpatrick Skin Type by your clinician.

Most changes are usually temporary and the skin will normally return to its natural colour within two to three months. Hypo-pigmentation (loss of colour) may not, however, resolve. A test patch may be performed at the pre-treatment consultation to assess your susceptibility to this. It tends to be more common in women with naturally dark skin. Protecting the treated area from the sun for at least two weeks before and after the treatment will help minimise any risk of pigment changes. Use a broad-spectrum sunscreen every day, regardless of weather. In some cases, despite our best efforts, the pigmentation may return. Other modalities may need to be used if this occurs.

Because the rejuvenation process involves the remodelling of matrix collagen, it may not be suitable for people who are susceptible to excessive scarring (e.g. keloids). Scar tissue is a rare side effect of IPL treatments and can be virtually eliminated as a risk by an experienced practitioner's knowledge of proper patient assessment and appropriate laser selection. However, it is important to avoid other procedures and treatments that induce collagen stimulation during the healing process, including cosmeceuticals.

SECTION 10:
TREATMENT OF VEINS

CHAPTER 31: SCLEROTHERAPY
CHAPTER 32: LASER SCLEROTHERAPY

It is fairly common as we age for the appearance of veins in our skin to become more prominent. One way this change manifests itself is in the development of what are known as 'spider veins'. Technically called 'telangiectasia', spider veins are clusters of very small veins, each one often no more than a millimetre or two wide, that spread out from a central point just under the surface of the skin. They can be quite knobbly or twisted in appearance and are usually dark blue or deep red in colour, and often resemble a road map or spider's web; hence the name.

Spider veins can develop on many different parts of the body (often on the face if excessively exposed to the sun), but most commonly they become visible on the legs. Besides the visual aspect, spider veins can also be a sign of associated skin problems, including ulcers, rashes such as eczema, and the formation of blood clots.

There are a number of factors that can influence the appearance of these blemishes, including changes in hormones, increased sedentariness, obesity, and simply the general ageing process, such as the reduced ability of the heart to pump blood down to the bottom of the body and back again.

You can take certain actions to try and prevent the development of spider veins – some of which are good practices for better health as you age anyway. For example, getting regular exercise, avoiding sitting down for long periods of time, and maintaining a healthy diet so that you do not become overweight or obese are all good steps to take. It is also recommended that you avoid wearing high-heeled shoes (at least not for extended periods of time), as the stress that is put on the legs by such footwear can inhibit the proper functioning of your veins. Support stockings can also be effective in limiting the appearance of spider veins.

However, despite taking preventative measures, spider veins can still appear. Fortunately, there are remedies available to treat them.

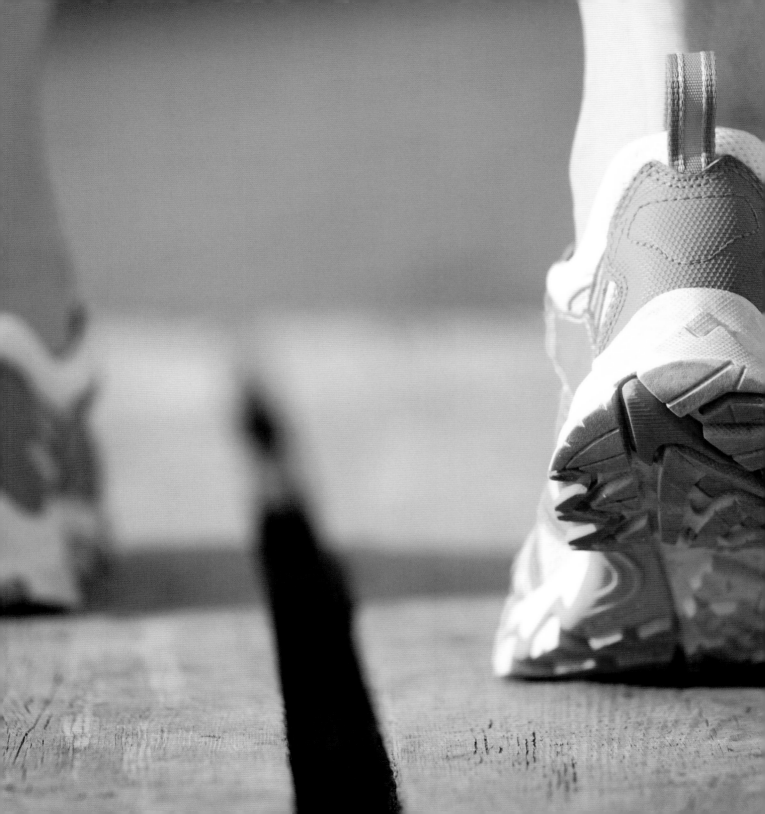

CHAPTER 31

SCLEROTHERAPY

Over 40 percent of women over the age of fifty have spider veins on their legs. Spider veins are chiefly a cosmetic problem but some women experience pain and discomfort from them. There are many different ways to improve the appearance of unsightly spider veins. Historically, the most popular has been sclerotherapy.

HOW DOES IT WORK?

Sclerotherapy involves injecting spider veins with a specially formulated and highly concentrated solution (known as a sclerosant). This chemical solution irritates the lining of the blood vessels, which causes the vessels to collapse (known as sclerosis). This prevents blood flow and means the unsightly vessel is far less visible. Over time a blood vessel that has undergone sclerosis will scar over and eventually disappear, along with the spider vein.

Many different substances can be used as sclerosants. The most popular and effective are detergents like polidocanol (POL) and sodium tetradecyl sulphate (STS). These have the advantage of being able to become foam in order to deal with bigger and central veins, and also can be used as a liquid for smaller jobs. Chemicals like glycerine are also widely used. Hypertonic saline can also be used in sclerotherapy.

Injections with scarring chemicals are not the only way to target unsightly veins or induce their sclerosis. Another way to get rid of small blood vessels is to cauterise them (dry them up) with a shot of electricity. This is often called electrocautery or electrosurgery (although there are no needles and no surgery). Essentially the low-level current from a Teflon-coated pinpoint electrode placed on the skin heats up the tissues directly under the point of contact. This causes the water to evaporate and the vessel underlying the needlepoint to collapse. It is quite effective for tiny superficial vessels or cherry spots, and it's relatively cheap, but electricity is not suitable for larger veins. It is also not perfectly selective and the surrounding skin risks getting damaged, causing problems with pigmentation, bleaching or scarring if too much electricity is applied.

WHO SHOULDN'T UNDERGO SCLEROTHERAPY?

Sclerotherapy injections are not generally recommended for women who are pregnant or breastfeeding. If you've had previous problems with clotting and blood disorders, then you should not undergo this procedure. During hot summer months, heat-induced dilation of blood vessels and inability to comply with wearing tight compression hose during recovery may also indicate that postponement of sclerotherapy to a later time is more appropriate.

Sclerotherapy in very overweight patients can also be difficult, as it is impossible to maintain adequate compression after the procedure to ensure blood vessels stay closed.

Some veins may just be too big to fix with sclerotherapy, and other techniques may be required, such as surgery or endovenous ablation.

WHAT CAN BE EXPECTED DURING AND AFTER SCLEROTHERAPY?

Sclerotherapy is a very simple process that can be performed at a practitioner's office or outpatient clinic. The procedure itself takes about 30 to 45 minutes, depending on the size and number of veins to be injected, and the extent of the treatment area.

Throughout the procedure, you will be lying on your back with your legs elevated. Before injecting, your practitioner will cleanse the skin over the target blood vessels with alcohol. Sometimes your practitioner will use an ultrasound device or transillumination machine with a light source to identify the best points for injection.

Sclerotherapy is relatively painless with minimal complications; therefore, anaesthesia is not usually necessary. However, some patients may want to use local anaesthesia or a numbing cream to minimise any discomfort as the veins are injected with the sclerosant solution.

The solution will be injected into the appropriate vein using a very fine needle. The practitioner will usually treat the largest and the deepest veins first, highest up your leg, before progressing to smaller ones further down. As many as ten injections may be performed for larger veins in one treatment session, while as many as fifty small injections may be used across a cluster of smaller veins.

RECOVERY AND AFTERCARE FOR SCLEROTHERAPY

After the treatment, you will be able to drive yourself home and return to your regular activities. However, one of the keys to a successful outcome is keeping the target area compressed with wraps or support hosiery for one to two weeks immediately following the injection. This puts pressure on the veins and holds them closed while the scarring that will keep them closed takes place.

Your practitioner will typically advise you to walk around and move your legs in order to prevent blood clots from forming and to increase blood flow to other veins. Ideally, walking should be done for at least 30 minutes every day, especially for the first few days after the procedure. However, you should avoid strenuous physical activities for a fortnight following your treatment.

Injection sites should be kept clean by regularly washing with mild soap and lukewarm water. Your skin may be sensitive to temperature for the first 48 hours or so after the treatment, so avoid taking hot baths or applying hot compresses to the injection sites. Sun exposure on the treated areas, as well as bed or fake tanning, should also be avoided for 48 hours after the treatment in order to avoid inflammation that may lead to permanent skin pigmentation.

Although significant discomfort is uncommon when using modern techniques and sclerosant solutions, if you do experience any mild pain, you can use paracetamol as required. Other medications such as aspirin, ibuprofen and NSAIDS should be avoided, as they may increase the risk of bruising or bleeding.

WHAT ARE THE RESULTS? HOW LONG WILL IT LAST?

In expert hands, sclerotherapy will be able to eliminate over 80 percent of the treated veins and produce excellent cosmetic results. Although there is an initial visible improvement, depending on the size of veins treated it takes three to six weeks for small veins and three to four months for large veins to fully disappear. Veins that respond to the solution usually do not reappear.

A follow-up visit with your practitioner is usually planned one to two months after the procedure to determine if any repeat treatments are needed. If it hasn't worked, the concentration, but not the volume, of sclerosant solution injected will be increased.

WHAT ARE THE POSSIBLE RISKS?

Sclerotherapy is a cheap, safe procedure that is relatively painless and has few complications. Some patients experience temporary but minor side effects, such as discomfort or bruising, raised red areas or small sores at the injection site, but these almost always quickly resolve themselves without additional treatment.

Between 10 and 30 percent of patients develop staining or brown spots along the course of the vein (known as hyperpigmentation), which may take several months to clear. Lasers can be used to help clear any pigmentation.

Sometimes when treating spider veins, new fine vessels may emerge after the treatment in a blush-like manner surrounding the treated area. This is known as matting. It is less common when experienced practitioners are doing the job, but it is likely in women on HRT and those who are overweight. However, experienced practitioners will usually be able to avoid causing it. Treatment for matting is usually not required since it will typically resolve itself over six to eight months.

On rare occasions, some of the injected solution doesn't end up in the vein where it is supposed to go, but leaks out into the skin (known as extravasation). All the chemicals used for sclerotherapy have the potential to harm non-targeted tissue if they make contact with it. This can be acutely painful, may wound the skin and can lead to blanching or ulceration. If a leak is detected at the time of the procedure, your practitioner may inject saline into the site to dilute the sclerosant, apply nitroglycerin paste and/or massage the area to spread the solution out as quickly as possible. Finally, by clotting a superficial leg vein there is a risk of the clot extending to affect deeper veins in the leg (known as deep vein thrombosis or DVT) or breaking free to affect the lungs (known as pulmonary embolism or PE). However, such risks are very minimal.

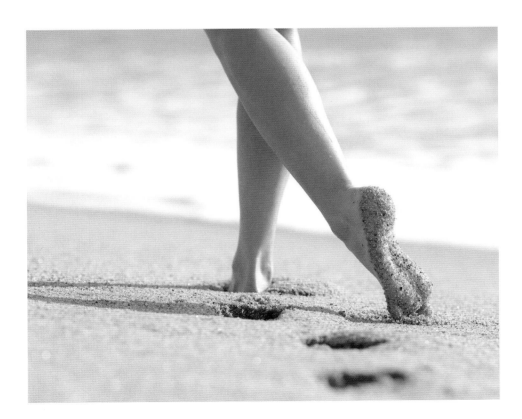

LASER SCLEROTHERAPY

There is a non-invasive alternative to sclerotherapy or surgery for getting rid of spider veins. Special lasers can selectively heat up and sclerose blood vessels. These are called vascular lasers, as they only work on blood vessels.

HOW DOES IT WORK?

All lasers work by shining light at a specific wavelength onto the skin, heating it up. The wavelength of the laser and its pulse frequency determines which cells it will heat up and at what depth. By tuning the frequency of a laser to a precise wavelength it is possible, for instance, to only heat up the red pigment in blood cells, the haemoglobin. This can help collapse unsightly blood vessels, while the surrounding skin is unaffected (as it does not absorb light at that wavelength).

The most common vascular lasers are argon lasers, potassium titanyl phosphate (KTP) lasers, yttrium-aluminium-garnet (Nd:YAG) lasers, copper vapour lasers, and pulsed dye lasers (PDL), which deliver a series of overlapping beams. The wavelength of the laser and the duration of each pulse can be selectively adjusted to suit the depth of the vein and its size. This takes a lot of skill and, like all areas of cosmetic medicine, and there is no one-size-fits-all approach. Vascular lasers are especially useful for getting rid of smaller spider veins matting (which occurs after sclerotherapy) and red spots (known as cherry angiomas). Obviously laser is also very useful for women who don't like needles or who are allergic or sensitive to some of the sclerosants used for injections.

It is sometimes not possible to treat larger veins non-invasively from the outside. The only way to selectively target such veins is to get the heat inside them. This is known as endovenous ablation. The most common procedures for this use laser or radiofrequency devices that are threaded inside the problem vein. On the end of the wire are electrodes that touch the walls of the vein. When in the right position these electrodes deliver energy that heats up the vein walls to around 120°C, but only to a depth of a few millimetres. This causes the vein to contract and shrink inward, and in most cases it will completely disappear within a month of treatment and seldom comes back. Because of the shallow depth of the procedure, only the vein wall is heated, and the rest of the skin is unaffected. This means that side effects from the procedure are minimal, and related largely to the puncture of the access vein. Nonetheless, this is not a simple procedure as it takes a lot of planning with ultrasound to track the target vein, and a surgical setup to ensure safe delivery. It tends, therefore, to be offered more by specialist vein clinics or by vascular and cosmetic surgeons.

WHO SHOULDN'T UNDERGO LASER SCLEROTHERAPY?

Spider veins on the legs are not as easy to treat with lasers as they are with injection sclerotherapy. This is because spider veins on the legs are generally deeper, larger and thicker than spider veins elsewhere, such as the face where lasers can be highly effective.

The big issue with laser therapies is that the skin pigment melanin can also absorb some laser energy and heat up at the same wavelengths that are used to destroy blood vessels. This means that lasers are not recommended for women with naturally dark or tanned skin, because of the risk of skin bleaching. Similarly, women treated with retinoids within the previous six months should avoid laser sclerotherapy because of the increased sensitivity of skin cells to all light, including laser. Anyone with a history of light-induced skin problems, or who is prone to scarring or vitiligo should not have vascular laser treatments. As with injection sclerotherapy, lasers are not generally recommended for women who are pregnant or breastfeeding, as the veins are often in a state of flux. Indeed, some (but not all) of the veins that become visible during pregnancy will disappear in the first six months after delivery. If you've had previous problems with clotting and blood disorders, then you should not undergo this procedure. During hot summer months, heat-induced dilation of blood vessels and an inability to comply with wearing tight compression hose during recovery may mean that postponement of treatment to a later time is appropriate. Some veins may be too big to fix with laser sclerotherapy alone, and other techniques may be required, such as surgery or endovascular ablation.

WHAT CAN BE EXPECTED DURING AND AFTER THE PROCEDURE?

Laser sclerotherapy is a simple procedure that can be performed at a practitioner's office or outpatient clinic. The procedure itself takes between 30 and 45 minutes, depending on the size and number of veins being treated. Throughout the procedure, you lie on your back with your legs elevated. A thin layer of water-based gel is applied to the skin's surface prior to treatment to make it easy to move the handpiece over the skin. The handpiece is then shone over the spider veins. Cooling is very important to reduce the risk of damage to overlying skin, so a cooling spray is used or the handpiece incorporates a cold-sapphire cooling mechanism. Often cooling starts before the laser procedure and continues after.

Each vessel is treated with a couple of passes of the handpiece to ensure complete coverage, signalled by the blue vessels becoming dark blue or the red vessels literally disappearing. The total procedure usually takes 10–15 minutes. Typically, a second or third treatment is required to complete the process, which can be performed at fortnightly intervals after the first procedure. Laser sclerotherapy usually causes a little discomfort. Topical anaesthetics can offset this but often other painkillers are required.

RECOVERY AND AFTERCARE

After the treatment, you will be able to drive yourself home and return to your regular activities. Your skin may be sensitive to temperature for the first couple of days after the treatment, so you should not take hot baths or apply hot compresses on the treatment sites. Often, a water-based moisturiser will be recommended for use over a couple of weeks following the procedure in order to ensure that the overlying skin remains healthy. Sun exposure on the treated areas, as well as bed or fake tanning, should also be avoided until the course of treatment is completed; this is to prevent any changes in skin pigmentations.

WHAT ARE THE RESULTS? HOW LONG WILL IT LAST?

Although it has the advantage of being non-invasive, laser sclerotherapy is generally not as effective a treatment for spider veins in the legs as injection sclerotherapy. The time it takes for the treated vein to disappear is also slower for laser than it is for injection sclerotherapy, and multiple treatments may be necessary to get the desired results. However, much also depends on the vessel size, colour and type of laser being used. For example, much better responses to laser are achieved for very small spider veins as opposed to larger veins. So treating small veins with laser can achieve comparable results to sclerotherapy and really small ones (like those associated with matting) are simply too small to inject so are best treated with lasers. Once the spider veins have collapsed they usually don't come back because the channels along which they ran have been obliterated.

WHAT ARE THE POSSIBLE RISKS OF LASER SCLEROTHERAPY?

Laser sclerotherapy on the legs is generally a very safe procedure, but it can be associated with some discomfort, more than with injection sclerotherapy. Lasers can also sometimes trigger changes in the pigmentation of the skin being treated, with either an increase (darkening) or decrease (bleaching) being observed, even when used on those with light skin. Some people also report changes in the texture of the skin after vascular laser therapy.

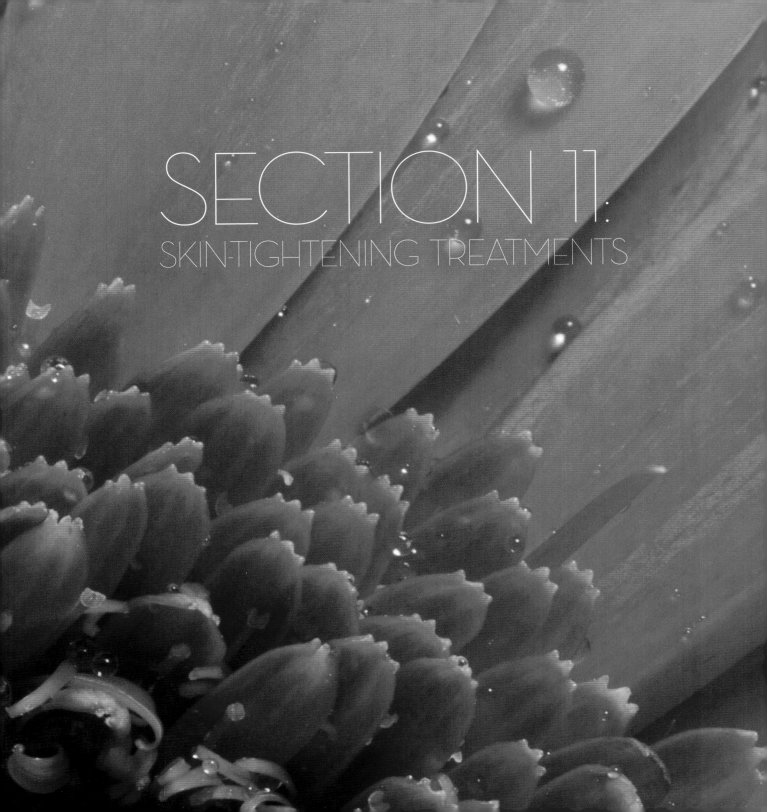

SECTION 11:
SKIN-TIGHTENING TREATMENTS

CHAPTER 33: RADIOFREQUENCY FOR SKIN TIGHTENING
CHAPTER 34: ULTRASOUND FOR SKIN TIGHTENING

There can be little doubt in the mind of any woman who looks in the mirror that as we age, our skin changes. It loses its smooth texture and, most of all, it begins to sag. There are many reasons for this, including the hormone changes we experience with the menopause. Other factors such as lifestyle, diet and the amount of exposure the skin has had to the damaging rays of the sun also play a part. If you smoke, the damage from free radicals in the skin cells can create unstable oxygen molecules that result in dry, dead-looking skin that has lost its tightness. But age, and the accompanying loss of elastin that helps to keep skin tight and smooth, is probably the biggest factor in skin losing its tautness.

As our skin loses elasticity, we see jowls develop, our cheeks become less full, and drooping begins to show around the eyelids. We see our face change from the full healthy rounded look of youth to one that sags in all the wrong places. In addition, other areas of our body such as our arms (particularly around the armpits) and our legs develop the same tendency.

Previously the only solution to these developments was to go 'under the knife' and get plastic surgery. However, that was often accompanied by long periods of painful recovery and possible side effects that could be devastating. Fortunately, today there are several non-invasive techniques to tighten sagging skin that have been shown to have remarkable results – without the pain, blood and danger of elective surgery.

Treatments such as radiofrequency and ultrasound – formerly just used by plastic surgeons to treat birthmarks and other skin abnormalities – as well as injectables and other skin resurfacing techniques such as laser and chemical peels have become well-documented and successful methods to tighten skin and restore its youthful elasticity.

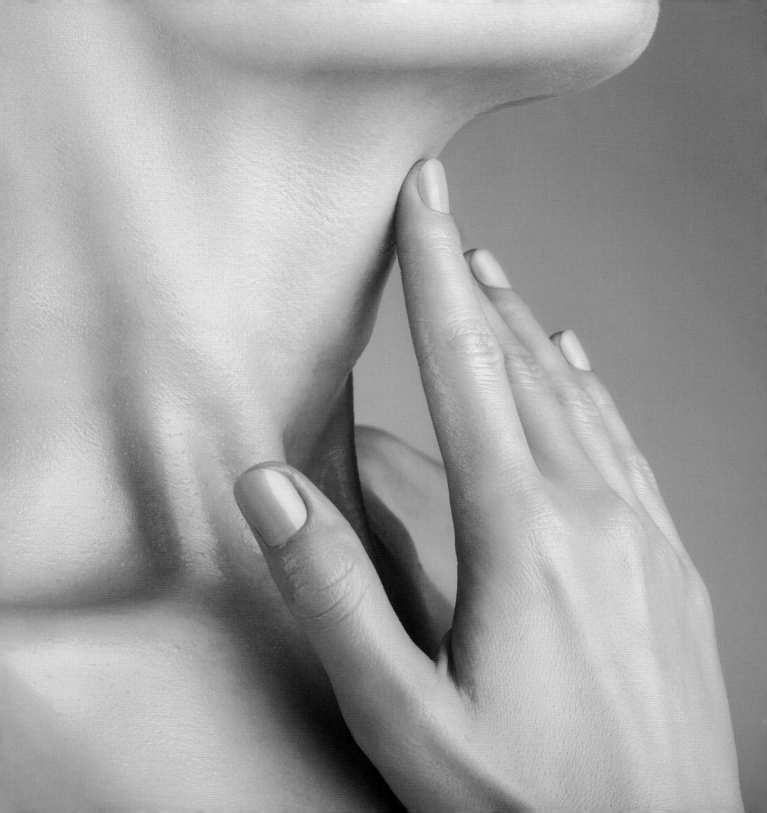

CHAPTER 33.

RADIOFREQUENCY FOR SKIN TIGHTENING

Radiofrequency energy is an exciting new way to target the deeper layers of the skin in a carefully controlled manner, without affecting the surface. Like laser photorejuvenation, radiofrequency works by heating the matrix proteins in the skin causing them to denature, contract and tighten. Like laser, radiofrequency procedures are often promoted as 'a non-surgical facelift' and used for treating skin laxity and sagging – on the chin, the folds around the nose, wrinkles and lines around the mouth and the forehead, and excess skin on the upper eyelid or bags under the eyes.

Our skin is resistant to the passage of electricity. As a result, it heats up when an electric current is passed through it. By doing this very gently, it is possible to heat the deep layers of the skin to between 65 and 75°C. At this temperature, the collagen fibres of the matrix denature and contract. This produces causes almost immediate tightening of the skin. At the same time, the outer surface of the skin is kept cool, so is unaffected by the process and remains completely intact.

Over the following few months, the heat-damaged matrix is progressively removed by the body and replaced with young, healthy collagen. Ultimately, this leads to stronger, firmer, smoother skin with a more youthful appearance.

The deep layers of the skin that heat up with radiofrequency can't be reached by conventional laser therapy. This means the effects of radiofrequency are different and synergistic to laser (with which it is often used in combination). In theory, this allows the laser to treat the outer part of the skin, while the radiofrequency component penetrates deeper into the skin for better and more complete results.

Other combination treatments are also used. For example, in combination with volumisers radiofrequency can be used to improve and augment the collagen responses; while in combination with botulinum toxin it helps to relax the muscle while the skin contracts.

Newer radiofrequency technologies have taken a leaf out of the laser book, with the development of fractional radiofrequency devices. As with laser, these devices treat only a fraction of the skin's area, allowing for more rapid healing with minimal side effects.

Radiofrequency produces better results in some people compared to others. For example, radiofrequency is far less effective in overweight people and in smokers. The tightening effect of radiofrequency may also be more marked in younger people. This is thought to be because the bonds that hold collagen together are more easily broken by heating young skin compared with older skin, where the collagen is less easily denatured by heating. Finally, radiofrequency works best for modest changes. Major sagging and deep lines will not be addressed by radiofrequency alone. It does have the advantage of being safe, quick and delivered in a single treatment, as well as avoiding the drawbacks of surgery, with its long recovery time and risk of complications. Radiofrequency can also be used on areas other than the face, to tighten bums, arms and thighs, for instance.

WHAT CAN I EXPECT DURING AND AFTER RADIOFREQUENCY TREATMENT?

No major preparation is required prior to radiofrequency treatment. It is recommended that you avoid taking warfarin, aspirin or anti-inflammatory drugs like NSAIDS (e.g. ibuprofen, ketoprofen) for one to two weeks before the procedure in order to reduce the risk of bruising. Some practitioners also recommend stopping vitamin E, ginseng, fish-oil tablets and herbal supplements that have anticoagulant effects for the same reason. Some also prefer their clients to stop taking oral contraceptives prior to the procedure, because of their effects on bleeding and clotting. Radiofrequency is generally not recommended for people with cardiac pacemakers or metal implants.

Radiofrequency treatment is performed as an outpatient procedure in a doctor's office or a private clinic. Depending on the treatment area, the procedure may take anywhere from 15 minutes to two hours. Treatments on the face typically last around 45 minutes, while procedures on other parts of the body may take up to an hour and a half, depending on the size of the area being treated.

Prior to a treatment, the area of skin that will be targeted is thoroughly cleansed. Eye protection is required for treatments around the eyes and if treating around the mouth, the teeth need to be kept cool (usually with a wet gauze placed between the teeth and the lips).

The practitioner will often apply a treatment grid as a guide. Coupling fluid is then applied generously to the areas to be treated, to facilitate the flow of electricity in the skin. The applicator probe is then placed in contact with the skin and calibrated to deliver exactly the right dose of energy for the skin area being treated. Once everything is set to go, a series of passes (usually three or four) are made over the area. At the same time, the skin is monitored for signs of tightening, redness or swelling (which are a sign that things are working).

Women undergoing the treatment often describe a brief sensation of heat, pinching or prickling, and a warming sensation similar to a facial massage. It's usually not necessary to apply topical numbing cream, administer local anaesthetic, or give oral pain medications, especially with newer devices that include forced air cooling of the skin surface. However, if pain is experienced, oral painkillers like paracetamol are usually preferred, because the area targeted is deeper than most topical creams can reach.

Some people may notice that their skin is tighter immediately after the treatment, while others see improvements after a few weeks. In most cases, results will appear gradually and the skin will continue to improve over several months, as the skin produces more collagen. The effects may last for up to one year after the treatment. While one treatment may be enough, most patients repeat their treatment after one or two years.

RECOVERY AND POSSIBLE SIDE EFFECTS OF RADIOTHERAPY TREATMENT

There's little or no downtime for recovery with radiofrequency treatments, so you can quickly return to your normal activities. It is common for a soothing restorative cream to be applied following the procedure and continued for several days. Makeup can be applied immediately after the treatment session, as the epidermis is unaffected.

Radiofrequency is a very safe treatment with only minor and temporary potential side effects. The most common issues are moderate discomfort during the procedure, and redness and swelling afterwards, which typically lasts for a couple of hours. If you feel uncomfortable, place a cold compress or an ice pack on the treated area to help reduce pain and swelling.

Radiofrequency can be used safely for patients of all skin types (it is said the treatment is 'colour blind') and is not normally associated with pigment changes in the skin, even in those prone to them.

Some people develop abrasions (known as crusting) in the treated area. These usually heal within three to four days. Occasionally some women experience temporary changes in sensation in the treated area, including itching or numbness. These symptoms are usually mild and typically resolve themselves completely within days.

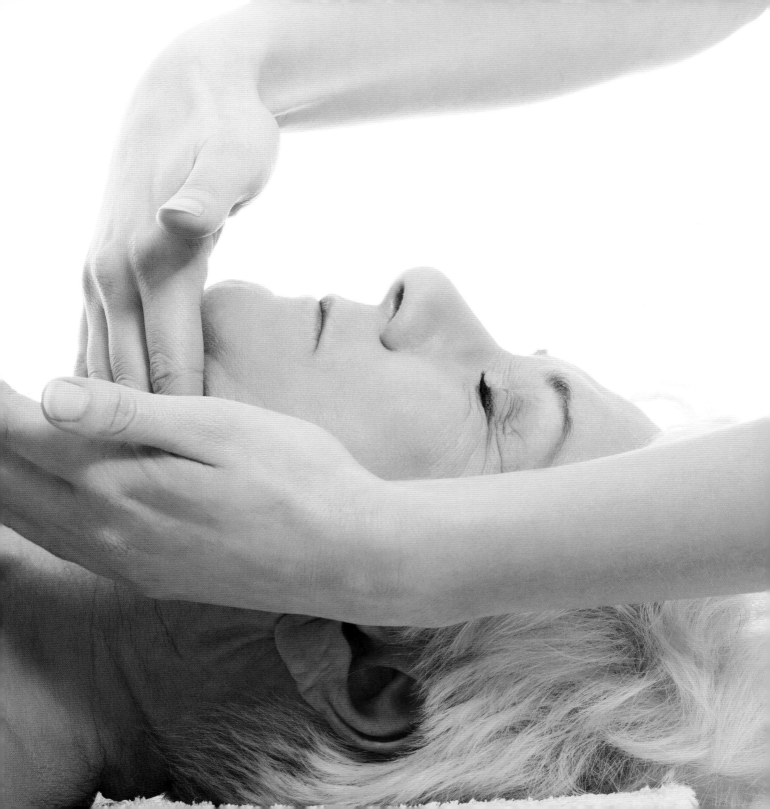

ULTRASOUND FOR SKIN TIGHTENING

Ultrasound is a technology that most people associate with medical imaging, like looking at a baby in utero. But the same technology can also be applied as a medical or cosmetic treatment. Blowing up stones in the kidney and treating injured muscles are clinical examples, while ultrasound selectively focused under the skin also can be used to break down underlying fat.

When used in cosmetic medicine, ultrasound devices deliver short pulses of focused acoustic energy in a concentrated high intensity beam to specific areas in or under the skin. For example, ultrasound waves can be focused at a specific energy and depth for the deep dermis, without damaging the overlying skin or underlying nerves. As with laser and radiofrequency, ultrasound causes controlled overheating of the matrix proteins in the skin dermis, and this causes the matrix collagen to contract and denature. The result is that the skin becomes visibly tighter and more elastic. Ultrasound is often marketed as a non-surgical facelift and used for treating chin sagging, folds around the nose, jowl and neck lift, wrinkles and lines around the mouth and the forehead, as well as excess skin on the upper eyelid.

Ultrasound also sets off an inflammatory response that sees the breakdown of old collagen and its replacement with healthy young collagen. This leads to stronger, firmer, smoother skin with a more youthful appearance.

On its own, its skin-tightening effects are more modest than surgery or other treatments such as injections or fillers. Consequently, ultrasound is more often used for making mild changes, or in combination with other treatments to achieve a more complete result. For example, it is used in combination with fillers to improve and augment the collagen responses with botulinum toxin, which relaxes the muscle while the skin contracts.

ULTRASONIC CAVITATION

Ultrasound can also be used to liquefy excess fat underlying the skin, which can then be sucked out. This is commonly known as ultrasonic cavitation or 'liposuction without surgery.' Sometimes a wetting solution is applied to help focus the ultrasound and dissolve the fat better. This is also known as VASER (which stands for vibration amplification of sound energy at resonance) and is a popular alternative or adjunct to liposuction, mesotherapy, cryo-sculpting or other fat-melting treatments.

Another use for ultrasound is extracorporeal pulse activation therapy (EPAT) also known as extracorporeal acoustic wave therapy (AWT), or shockwave therapy. It is mostly used for the treatment of muscle or tendon injuries. However, it can also be used to stimulate remodelling of ageing skin, with increased synthesis of collagen and elastin. It is also popular for the treatment of cellulite.

WHAT TO EXPECT DURING ULTRASOUND THERAPY?

No major preparation is required prior to ultrasound treatment. It is recommended that you avoid taking warfarin, aspirin or anti-inflammatory drugs like NSAIDS (e.g. ibuprofen, ketoprofen) for one to two weeks before the procedure in order to reduce our risk of bruising. Some practitioners also recommend stopping vitamin E, ginseng, fish-oil tablets, and herbal supplements with anticoagulant effects for the same reason. Some doctors also prefer their clients stop taking oral contraceptives prior to the procedure, because of its effects on bleeding and clotting.

Depending on the treatment area, the procedure may take anywhere from 15 minutes to two hours. Treatments on the face typically takes around 45 minutes, while treatments on other parts of the body may take up to an hour and a half, depending on the size of the area being treated.

The practitioner will apply a treatment grid to the skin as a guide. The procedure involves holding a treatment tip (usually between half and three quarters of an inch wide) over the skin while the device releases the ultrasound probe underneath the epidermis. The treatment tip may pass over the skin several times.

When used for skin tightening, there is no point in applying topical numbing cream as the treatment targets deeper into the tissues. Practitioners will typically use oral pain medications or nitrous oxide to alleviate any pain. This is not for the faint hearted, as the procedure can be quite uncomfortable, depending on the area being treated.

There's little or no downtime for recovery after ultrasound. It is common for a soothing restorative cream to be applied following the procedure, and continued for several days. Makeup can be applied immediately after the treatment session, as the epidermis is unaffected.

Do not use hot water for at least two days when showering or bathing, as the treated skin may be more sensitive to temperature immediately after the treatment.

Results vary from patient to patient. Some people may notice that their skin is tighter immediately after the treatment while others see improvement only after a few weeks. The tightening effect of ultrasound may be more marked in younger people. This may be because the bonds that hold collagen together are more easily broken by heating in young skin. In most cases, results will appear gradually and the skin will continue to improve over several weeks and months as it produces more collagen. The effects may last for up to one year after the treatment. While one treatment may be enough, most patients repeat the treatment annually.

When used to treat fat and reduce our waistline, ultrasound can generally achieve reductions of about one dress size over a couple of months, with most of this loss observed within the first few weeks.

WHAT ARE THE POTENTIAL SIDE EFFECTS OF ULTRASOUND THERAPY?

Ultrasound is a safe treatment, usually with only minor and temporary side effects. The most common side effects are moderate discomfort during the procedure, and skin redness that typically lasts for one to two hours after the treatment. Your skin may be slightly pink or mildly swollen after the treatment, but this typically subsides after a few hours. Placing a cold compress or an ice pack on the treated area can help reduce pain and swelling if you experience discomfort. Some women notice temporary changes in sensation in the treated area, including itching or numbness. Such symptoms are usually mild and resolve completely in a few days. Rarely, overly aggressive or inexperienced treatments may lead to burns, indentations, scars or changes in pigmentation. These side effects are unlikely to happen with experienced practitioners.

SECTION 12:
CELLULITE AND FAT LOSS TREATMENTS

CHAPTER 35: CRYOSCULPTING FOR FAT LOSS
CHAPTER 36: ULTRASOUND FOR TREATMENT OF CELLULITE AND FAT LOSS
CHAPTER 37: RADIOFREQUENCY FOR FAT LOSS

One key change that occurs in our body as we age is the amount of body fat and its location. This has major implications for our health as well as our appearance.

Fat loss below the skin can leave areas looking hollow, especially under the eyes, and at the cheeks, chin and temples. But too much fat can also affect our appearance.

It tends to accumulate on the brow, jaws, under the chin, and on the neck, making an older face appear 'squared off' or 'unbalanced', compared to the defining arcs, lines and angular shape of our youth. In other areas fat can squeeze up and into connective tissue layers of the dermis, producing unsightly cellulite.

The obvious solution is to reduce fat under our skin. This can be achieved through weight loss programs, including exercise, diet and other lifestyle changes. But this is a gradual process and even with commitment it can be difficult to achieve and sustain. In particular, cellulite, muffin tops, and other specific fatty deposits can be hard to budge. But there are solutions.

Fat can be removed surgically with liposuction, which literally sucks up clusters of fat cells from under the skin. One of the most popular cosmetic surgeries, it is widely used for excess fat in the tummy (love handles/muffin tops), buttocks, hips, upper arms and thighs. It can even be used to treat cankles. But surgery has major costs and risks, including pain, the requirement of anaesthetic, bruising, scarring and considerable downtime for recovery.

Today we have procedures to remove fat from under the skin without breaking the skin – or the budget. These procedures, known medically as lipolysis or lipoplasty, include fat sculpting, contouring, or 'liposuction without surgery'. In each case they literally break up fat cells, leaving, using radio waves, ultrasound or extreme cold.

When used to treat fat around the waist, contouring can generally achieve a reduction of about one dress size over a couple of months. Lipolysis won't get rid of all the fat from our bodies, and we still need to watch what we eat and exercise more. But it can get us looking how we want to quickly, while our diet and lifestyle catches up.

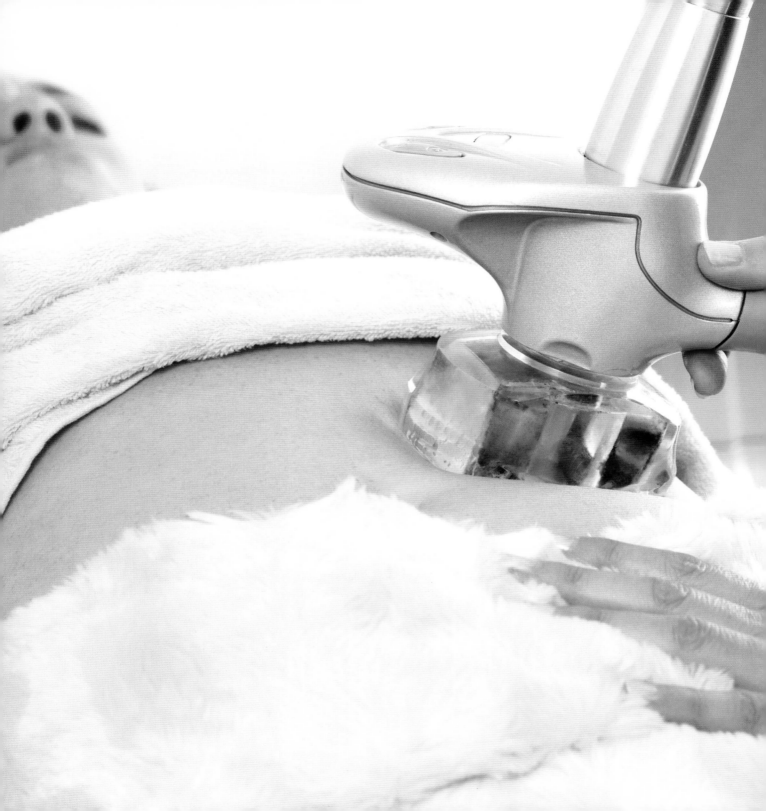

CHAPTER 35

CRYOSCULPTING FOR FAT LOSS

Cold temperatures can also be used to treat unwelcome fat deposits deep under the skin (a procedure known as cryolipolysis or coolsculpting). One story has it that this was discovered by accident after some women who had been horse riding out in the freezing cold developed red and inflamed thighs, and their cellulite suddenly disappeared – fat was literally getting frozen off their thighs.

WHAT TO EXPECT DURING THE TREATMENT

It is thought that fat is just a bit more sensitive to the cold than the rest of the skin. So if you apply exactly the right amount of cold temperature to the skin to freeze the fat, but not kill the skin above it (which is what happens in frostbite), only the fat will disappear. This is a delicate business and must be done be an expert practitioner.

Most cryosculpting makes use of a strong vacuum placed onto the skin to suck the skin (and its underlying fat) into a cup which is then chilled to around 50C for 30–60 minutes. This external suction on the skin is not liposuction, which is a surgical procedure where a vacuum is placed under our skin and sucks away the fat.

When undergoing the procedure, it is recommended that you refrain from taking aspirin or any other blood thinning medication for two weeks before the procedure. This will help to reduce any risks for bruising when the skin is sucked up into the vacuum cup. This is a very gentle procedure that takes place while you are lying down. The area where the treatment will take place will be thoroughly washed before the treatment and it is recommended that you do not wear perfume or cologne on the day of the treatment.

Many patients feel a cold sensation but cryotherapy is not usually painful. You can expect to return for several treatments to get the best possible results, as the effects are incremental in nature.

IS CRYOTHERAPY FOR EVERYONE?

While it is true that cryosculpting works well for many people, it is best for mild changes and those last few kilos around problem areas such as the tummy, buttocks or around the hips. It won't be as effective for people who are very overweight or who have more severe changes as a result of fat in their skin.

RECOVERY AND AFTERCARE

There may be transient discomfort during and immediately after the procedure. If the treated area of skin is exposed to very cold temperatures, sometimes you'll experience bruising and/or swelling as blood returns to the treated area as it warms up.

It is usually recommended that patients drink plenty of water for the first 24 hours after the procedure; this helps the body to eliminate the waste created by the procedure. Following a healthy diet and exercise routine can also help give the best possible results.

POSSIBLE SIDE EFFECTS OF CRYOTHERAPY

Cryotherapy can sometimes affect the pigmentation of the area being treated. The pigment producing cells (melanocytes) are particularly sensitive to the cold, even in low doses. When melanocytes are gone, colour is lost permanently. This is not a problem for fair skinned women, but it does mean that cryotherapy in women with dark skin should generally be avoided. Dark skinned women are also more prone to the opposite problem, where cryotherapy can transiently cause increased pigmentation of the treated area; this can last for several months. Cryotherapy can also cause permanent hair loss in the treated area.

CHAPTER 36
ULTRASOUND FOR TREATMENT OF CELLULITE AND FAT LOSS

Ultrasound is a technology that most people associate with medical imaging, like looking at a baby in utero. But the same technology can also be applied as a medical or cosmetic treatment. Blowing up stones in the kidney and treating injured muscles are clinical examples, while ultrasound selectively focused under the skin also can be used to break down underlying fat.

HOW DOES ULTRASOUND WORK FOR WEIGHT LOSS?

The principle is pretty simple. Ultrasound is a sound wave emitted at very high frequencies. When delivered at a specific energy and depth it selectively vibrates fat cells, causing them to heat up. This heat actually makes the fat cells break down, and this turns the fat cells into a liquid that the body can reabsorb quite readily.

The treatment is usually done with two paddles. They are held a few inches above the skin and moved over the area being treated in turn. The first paddle prepares the body for absorbing the destroyed fat cells by massaging the lymph system near to where the fat cells are being removed. The second paddle then sends out the sound waves and breaks the fat cells down. The first paddle is then passed over the area again, to direct the liquid from the broken fat cells towards the closest lymph nodes. They will then reabsorb this liquid into the body, a natural function for these organs.

This application is sometimes known as VASER (which stands for vibration amplification of sound energy at resonance).

WHAT TO EXPECT DURING THE TREATMENT?

There is no pre-treatment preparation required for an ultrasound session. The entire treatment takes anywhere between half an hour and two hours depending on the area being treated. Typically, you will lie for the treatment. A thin layer of gel will first be applied over the area of skin to be treated, then the paddles are moved over the skin to apply the ultrasound. You may feel a little bit of heat while the procedure is taking place. Some have compared the heat from the wand to the experience of having hot rock treatments at a massage; localised heat that is quite warm but not excessive.

The procedure is usually painless. There are a few areas of the skin, however, where some slight discomfort may be felt. If the treatment is being done in an area of the body where a large bone is nearby, such as the thigh, there might be a brief moment of intense heat as the paddles pass close to the bone, as when the ultrasound waves hit the bone they will bounce back, generating extra heat. That will pass quickly, especially if you let the practitioner know you feel the heat. Outside of this, the treatment is simply a series of warm sensations that doesn't produce any pain.

IS ULTRASOUND FOR EVERYONE?

This treatment is best suited to patients who are otherwise healthy and not greatly overweight. The ideal candidate will have already used exercise and a healthy diet to achieve a near optimal weight – the ultrasound is then used to target a few problem areas. It works best when the treatment areas are small and well defined, such as a pouchy belly after having a baby or sagging skin under the chin after going through menopause.

RECOVERY AND AFTERCARE

Because it is a non-invasive technique there are minimal side effects when it comes to ultrasound treatments. A small amount of inflammation or redness may remain for a few hours after the treatment, but that is simply the body responding to the heat produced during the procedure and it will soon dissipate.

It is recommended that patients drink plenty of water for the first 24 hours after the procedure to help the body to eliminate the waste created by the process. Following a healthy diet and exercise routine can also be beneficial and give the best results.

WHAT RESULTS CAN YOU EXPECT FROM ULTRASOUND TREATMENT?

The results are incremental, although improvements should be visible within the first two or three treatments. This means you will see a little change with each treatment, and will need between eight and ten treatments to get optimal results. It is recommended that the treatments be performed at two-week intervals to give the body time to heal and flush all of the unwanted fat cells that have been destroyed completely out of the body.

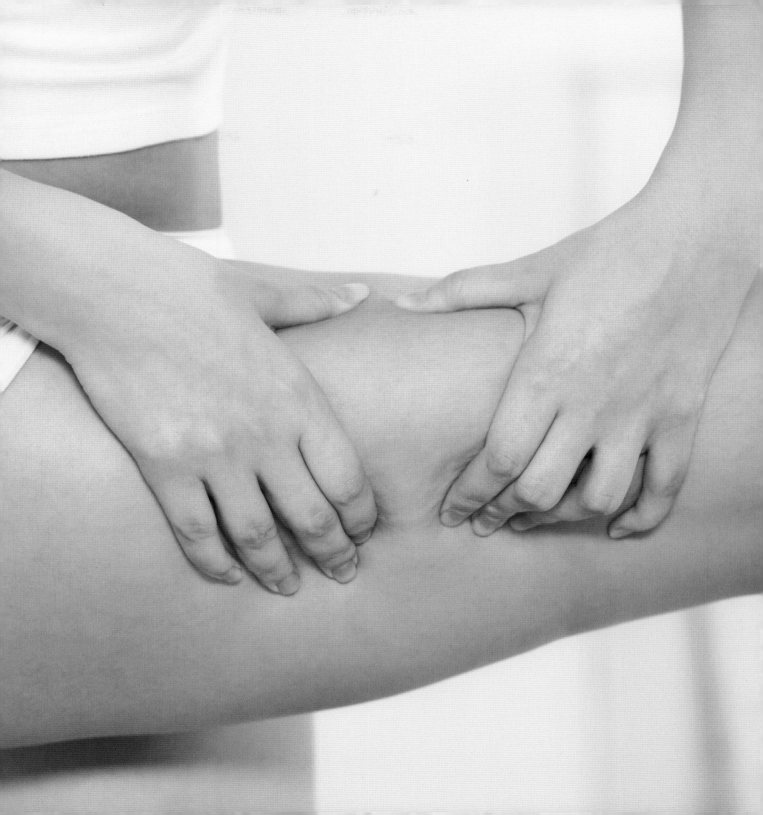

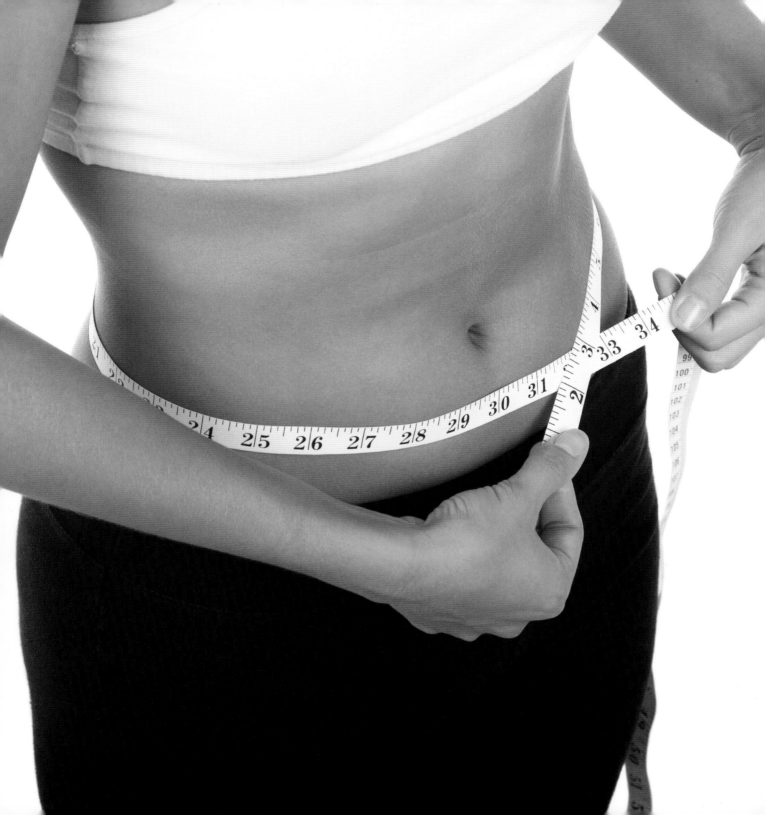

CHAPTER 37

RADIOFREQUENCY FOR FAT LOSS

Radiofrequency waves can also be used to break down unwanted fat tissues in the body. Unlike freezing or ultrasound, radiofrequency treatments can target larger areas at single time, making them ideal for areas such as the buttocks or for when a greater part of the tummy needs work.

However, it can also be targeted successfully for smaller areas giving it a greater versatility than most fat reduction techniques. As with the two previous treatments discussed, radiofrequency is a great tool for reducing pockets of stubborn fat that cannot be eliminated through diet and exercise.

HOW DOES RADIOFREQUENCY WORK?

The principle of radiofrequency treatments is very similar to ultrasound in that it uses radio waves to create heat in targeted fat cells. It usually involves a combination of both unipolar and bipolar radio frequencies. The heat is created when the radio waves are introduced at a subdermal level, identifying the fat cells via their water content. The radio waves can then zero in on these fat cells, and the high frequency of the waves causes vibrations in the cells that heat them up, resulting in them shrinking and then breaking down. The resulting cells are then easily absorbed into the body, eliminating the fat cells right at their source.

WHAT TO EXPECT DURING THE TREATMENT?

It is recommended that the patient refrain from taking aspirin or any other blood thinning medication for two weeks before the procedure. This will help to reduce the risk of bruising. It is also recommended that patients not wear perfume or cologne on the day of the treatment. Radiofrequency is a very gentle procedure that takes place while the patient is lying down. The area where the treatment will be applied is washed thoroughly prior to commencement.

A wand or similar device is held over the target area about an inch above the skin. Several passes are made over the treatment area in order to create and maintain the best possible temperature for the procedure. Many patients feel a slight tingling sensation, similar to what you might feel if an annoying child pestered you by snapping a rubber band on your skin over and over.

At the same time that these radio waves are heating up the fat cells, they are also helping to promote blood flow to the area for fast healing. This natural by-product of the procedure will also create a healthier skin tone because of the increased blood flow around the treated area. Expect to return for several treatments to get the best possible results, as the effects are incremental in nature.

IS RADIOFREQUENCY FOR EVERYONE?

While it is true that radiofrequency treatments can be used to treat a larger area of skin than the more narrowly focused ultrasound, they are still not intended for anyone who is grossly overweight. This treatment works best for someone who finds themselves unable to get rid of those last ten pounds around problem areas such as the tummy, buttocks or around the hips.

This is also not recommended for anyone who has had problems with blood clots or any other type of blood disorder, because of the increased blood flow during treatment. Radiofrequency treatments of any type are not recommended if the patient has a pacemaker or any metal implants. Those who wear braces on their teeth should avoid treatments of the face.

RECOVERY AND AFTERCARE

The recovery time is very short for radiofrequency treatments that target cellulite and fat reduction. The patient may notice a slight swelling in the first 24 hours or so after the treatment, and a warm sensation on the skin in the treated area. This is normal and should disappear within the first day, if not within the first few hours after treatment. A very small percentage of patients may feel an itching sensation for a day or two, but this will also quickly disappear.

An ice pack can be placed on the treated area if it makes the patient more comfortable, but all patients should be able to return to work the same day with no obvious after effects. Some patients may want to apply a soothing cream if they are particularly sensitive to heat or discomfort. Makeup can be worn the same day as the treatment.

It is recommended that patients drink plenty of water for the first 24 hours after the procedure to help the body eliminate the waste created by the procedure. Following a healthy diet and exercise routine can also be beneficial and help to give the best possible results.

WHAT RESULTS CAN YOU EXPECT FROM RADIOFREQUENCY TREATMENT?

As stated earlier, the results of radiofrequency treatment for fat reduction is incremental and requires several treatments. It is generally recommended that between three to six bi-weekly treatments be planned to get the best results. While fat reduction and smoother skin does result from the procedure, you should not expect drastic changes overnight.

The goal of most radiofrequency fat reduction treatments is to eliminate small areas that have been giving the patient trouble over the previous year or so. This can mean slowly dissipating those 'love handles' or helping that tummy pouch to melt away. It does not mean that thirty years of packing on the weight will be sloughed off in a week or two.

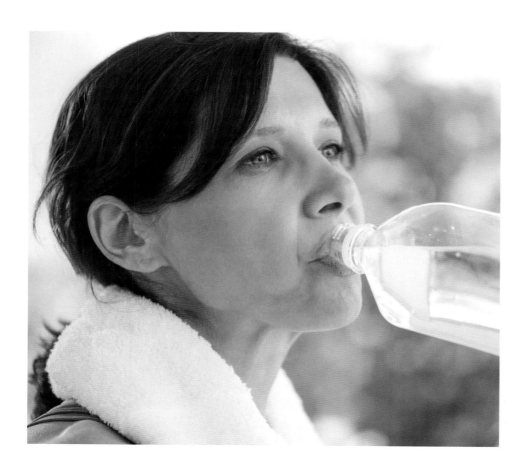

SECTION 13

MAKING AN INFORMED DECISION

CHAPTER 38: CHOOSING A PRACTITIONER

When it comes to treatments for achieving younger looking skin, it's not enough just to choose the right procedure; finding the right practitioner is also a critical decision if you want to achieve the best results.

A big part of this will be your relationship with the practitioner. Remember these are, after all, medical treatments. This means you want someone who knows the skin area well, has done plenty of treatments before, and can talk knowledgably and comfortably with you about your treatment options. Keep in mind that, with the right practitioner, you will have an expert to help you explore all your options. Too many patients first choose a procedure or a product then go with the first person they find who advertises that treatment. However, the real expertise is in how a procedure is performed or how a product is applied.

Of course, you shouldn't just rely on the word of the practitioner when making a decision. The internet can be a good source of information, but remember that when it comes to ratings and review sites, there is not verification system, so exaggerations – both positive and negative – are common.

Arguably better methods of getting information are to talk to your friends and see if they have had any experiences with practitioners they would recommend, and to ask your GP about who might be a good person to refer to.

But even with this guidance, you should always meet with a practitioner before deciding to undergo a treatment with them. Talk about your goals; discuss their successes and their failures. A good practitioner will be willing to talk about what they do when things go wrong as well as when they go right. Such discussions will help you to discover the practitioner that has practices in synch with your goals. Together you can define how the pathway to those goals will be created.

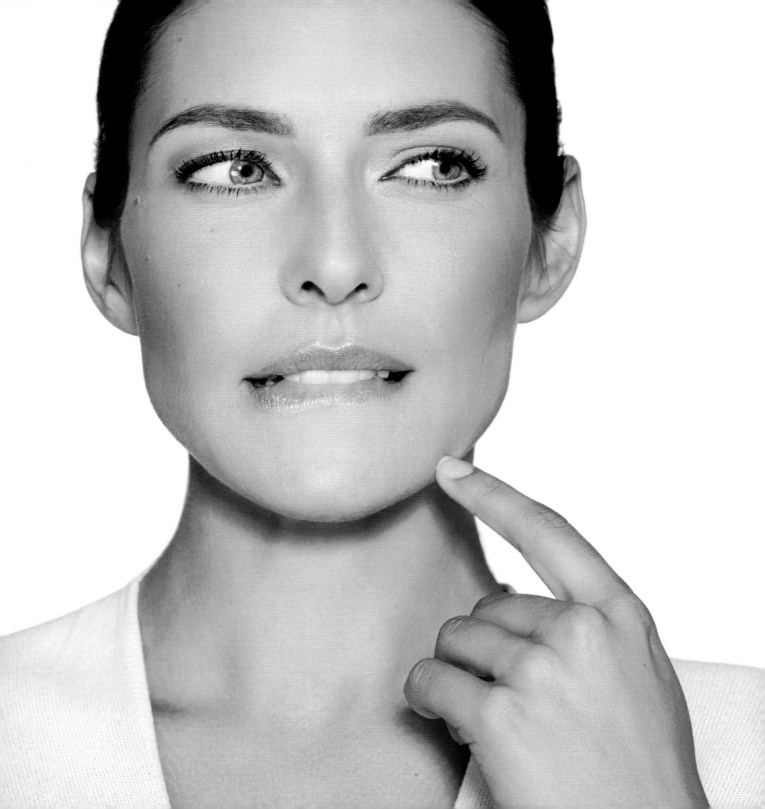

CHOOSING A PRACTITIONER

Cosmetic procedures should be performed by trained medical practitioners or nurses. Most cosmetic procedures are performed in specialised cosmetic medicine clinics, based around specific procedures or technologies, like laser or fat sculpting clinics. Many of these clinics offer both medical and surgical procedures, which will usually be delivered by different specialists within each clinic. Today, some general practitioners also offer a range of cosmetic procedures, such as anti-wrinkle injections and fillers. Here are some things to consider when looking for an appropriate practitioner.

CHECK TRAINING

The best practitioners are those who perform a procedure every day, have done it many times, and who have the familiarity and adaptability to give you a treatment that is best suited to your skin. Their skills are developed through years of formal education and training. Until recently, cosmetic medicine was not a significant part of the training of any of the long-established medical colleges. Practitioners who specialise in this field have usually trained privately or obtained practical experience in clinics. All practitioners should welcome questions regarding professional experience, qualifications, practice experience and their facilities.

The sole focus of the Australasian College of Cosmetic Surgery (ACCS), however, is cosmetic medical practice and it is generally regarded as the premier educational body in cosmetic medicine and surgery. Fellows of the Cosmetic Physicians College of Australia must meet stringent criteria to be admitted to the ACCS, and are typically among of the most experienced cosmetic physicians in Australia. The Australasian College of Cosmetic Medicine (ASCM) and other colleges offer training in some cosmetic procedures. For example, the Australasian College of Phlebology offers training in sclerotherapy. The Australian Medical Council (AMC) has recently begun considering cosmetic medical practice as a medical specialty, which is a precursor to establishing a specialist college to oversee training and practise.

CHECK PROFESSIONAL MEMBERSHIP

All the best practitioners are certified and members of professional agencies that give support as well as training in the latest techniques in cosmetic medicine, to ensure the delivery of the best results with the least side effects. Some practitioners, however, think they can go it alone. They may be certified in another specialty but not the one you are considering, or they may not be certified by one of the appropriately credentialed agencies. Such practitioners should be approached with caution. Cosmetic medicine is moving rapidly, with innovations, new technology and synergism between different approaches constantly evolving. It really pays to be up to date.

The Australasian College of Cosmetic Surgery (accs.org.au), the Cosmetic Physicians Society of Australasia (CPSA) (cosmeticphysicians.org.au) and the Australasian College of Cosmetic Medicine (ASCM) (acam.org.au) can all provide details on practitioners with expertise in cosmetic medicine. The Australian Health Practitioner Regulation Agency website (ahpra.gov.au) provides a list of registered health care and medical practitioners in Australia. Check the Australian Society of Plastic Surgeons at (plasticsurgery.org.au) to review a practitioner's qualifications, registration details and specialties.

PROMOTIONAL ACTIVITIES AND ADVERTISING

Cosmetic practitioners offering cosmetic procedures make use of different advertising sources, such as magazines, newspapers, TV, celebrity endorsements and the internet. The purpose of these advertisements is to sell, so the validity of any claims of success cannot be relied upon. Always seek to verify the information being presented from independent sources.

LISTING AND RANKING ON WEBSITES

Be careful on this one. Certain websites list the 'top leading cosmetic practitioners' without verifying the information. These sites can be misleading and the site owners may be getting referral fees, an incentive to put the practitioner with the highest referral fee in the top spot. There are no existing standards being followed when ranking the practitioners.

TALK TO THEM

The most important thing to do when considering a practitioner is to go and check them out. Make an appointment to meet the practitioner and see what they can offer. Medicine is also an art, not just a science. If you find someone who is interested in the unique characteristics of your skin, then you are most of the way there. Your relationship with your cosmetic practitioner will not be a one-off fling, but a long-term commitment. Choose someone with whom you can make that commitment.

Before you consult a practitioner, it's a good idea to make a list of questions. No matter how trivial they sound, it's your right to ask questions, and it's the practitioner's responsibility to answer them in a manner you can understand.

It is important to meet the prospective practitioner during the initial consultation. There are times when other members of the clinic may see you first, before the physician. These healthcare providers are mainly tasked with educating patients and conducting routine physical examinations. Although they can answer some of your questions, it's imperative to actually meet the practitioner who will perform the procedure. Don't settle for less. Find out as much as you can. The initial consultation is also the right time to address any questions, fears and concerns.

Convey your expectations and goals up front. Photos are a great way to let the cosmetic practitioner know what you see as the problem and how you would like your face to look after an intervention.

In addition, pay attention to the rapport you have with this professional. You will need to be able to communicate clearly to each other to get the result you want. You will need to be able to put your trust in this person, so ask yourself if you feel comfortable talking to them. Do they listen to you and respond to your questions? Even if your best friend can't sing their praises highly enough, that doesn't mean they are the right practitioner for you. If that connection, trust and ability to communicate isn't there, move on.

ASK QUESTIONS CONCERNING THE PROCEDURE

What kind of procedures and treatments are available? Where do you start and why? How often should you have treatments? Are you really a good candidate for the procedure you are thinking of having? If not, can you do something to be a good candidate in the future? How long is the recovery period? What follow-up treatment is best? Will there be a need for touch-ups?

These are just some of the queries you might have with regard to a particular treatment. Discuss the chances for unwanted things like pain, days off work, ugly changes in the skin and other complications, and ask how you can control or minimise them.

Good practitioners should have a history of successful treatments that they are happy to discuss with you. Ask for portfolio photos of other people who have had the same kind of procedures. What kind of results did they get from being treated by this practitioner?

DISCUSS YOUR HEALTH AND FAMILY HISTORY

Be completely open with your potential practitioner about any health concerns, medical issues, medications and other factors that could influence your suitability for a treatment, such as whether you smoke or are trying to become pregnant.

DISCUSS THE TOTAL COST

Ask about the practitioner's fee, and relevant fees for anaesthesia, follow-ups, post-procedural tests if needed, and supplies. Discuss financing options and payment plans. You want to know exactly what the treatment will cost before committing to it. Most cosmetic procedures are not covered by health insurance, but a few are, so always check your policy.

Remember, cheapest is not the always the best – or safest – option. For example, some practitioners use less botulinum toxin units than required; this cuts the cost but also compromises the results. Shop for quality; if you base your decisions solely on price, it's likely that you won't be satisfied with the results.

HOW MUCH SHOULD IT COST?

Every well-informed cosmetic procedure decision comes with a price tag. If you've been saving up for months or years for a cosmetic intervention, you probably know that your finances will certainly make a big impact on our decision. It will help you decide on a clinic or cosmetic practitioner. In fact, your financial status will affect whether or not you can go ahead with a procedure at all.

Prices will vary from case to case, depending on the type of treatment, the size of the area that needs to be treated, the geographical location of the clinic and the practitioner's fees. The large number of providers and competition in the industry means that prices have fallen significantly over the past decade or so and appear set to continue to fall. The internet can be good source of pricing information, but many clinics don't always indicate the specific prices on their websites (for fear of scaring you away!).

Clinics are business operations; bear this in mind at all times. They will try to get every opportunity to sell you their 'goods.' There's nothing wrong with this as long as they respect your rights as a consumer. You are not obligated to buy every pair of shoes you try on every time you go shopping. Shopping for a cosmetic procedure works the same way. If it doesn't fit, and the price is not right, don't buy it.

Listen to your gut. It may not be an exact science, but don't doubt your instincts. Do not sacrifice your health for a few dollars of savings.

GREAT EXPECTATIONS

Find a practitioner who can provide a realistic assessment of the benefits and risks of a treatment. Have a discussion about the options and about any complications that can arise with each. Understand that sometimes expectations exceed what is possible, even for the best practitioner. But a frank discussion of what to expect, and whether the goals are achievable will give you a good grounding from which to start the ball rolling.

If a practitioner gives you unrealistic guarantees of perfect outcomes, then you should look more closely at the whole deal. Complications and risks are always involved, no matter how common a procedure might be. Anyone who guarantees perfect outcomes every time is untrustworthy.

UNDER PRESSURE

Undertaking a cosmetic procedure is an important decision, but it is not emergency surgery. There is no reason to feel pressured into making a decision on the spot. Take your time, and if you feel as though you are being put under undue pressure, back away.

This includes any pressure you have put on yourself to have this treatment. It will have a lasting effect on you and your body. In the end it is important that you treat your body with respect, and that you have a sense that your practitioner has that same sense of respect. Never let any sense of urgency from you or anyone else push you into making a decision. If you are not sure, it can always wait.

INDIVIDUALISATION

A practitioner should take a comprehensive medical history and conduct a physical examination, not just look at the target area of the skin. They should see you as a unique person with your own goals and desires. It is important that this be the cornerstone of your relationship with them. When it is, even complications can be solved because they will have the level of trust needed to arrive at the right solutions for you as an individual.

APPENDIX:
KATE MARIE (AUTHOR) STORY

MY AGEING FACE

We all age; it is a fact of life. But if there is one thing I have become more aware of as I grow older, it is that we don't all age in the same way or at the same pace. Nature doesn't always play favourites or reward you for good behaviour, so it can be annoying to see how we can be 'penalised' looks-wise despite our good health practices. Weight is a prime example. If you are overweight, then the signs of ageing aren't always so apparent on your face – that extra layer of fat often gives our faces a smoother appearance.

I'm lucky to have a high metabolism, and I've worked hard to be lean and fit, but as a consequence I can look a bit skeletal, particularly around my eyes and cheeks. While it may be true that staying slim is healthy, I am not ready to look like a skeleton. Luckily there are solutions to this and so I have been using fillers and other treatments to encourage as much collagen growth in my skin as possible. I have used fillers to fill out hollow areas on a regular basis in conjunction with platelet-rich plasma (PRP). I'm not attached to any one brand as have tended to go along with the products recommended by my various trusted practitioners. I've tended to be a bit of a guinea pig though and I have made mistakes by being a bit too experimental at times. For instance, I've now got nodules in the back of my hands as a result of bad advice from one of the reps from a well-known filler company. The filler companies don't tend to take responsibility for these kinds of mistakes and usually claim that the results are dependent on the practitioner's skill.

The other downside of a high metabolism means that some products seem to disappear relatively quickly. No one enjoys the sensation of needles, even the tiny ones used for injections and I am no exception. By using a longer acting treatment I also avoid going through the discomfort of the treatment more times than necessary. There is no such thing as a completely pain-free treatment when it comes to injections, and while facial injections are certainly not my favourite way to spend time, the results make the (minor) pain worthwhile.

AGEING LIPS

I have to confess, most of my family missed out when they were handing out discernible lips. When I first started doing cosmetic treatments and had my lips plumped a bit, I thought I'd died and gone to heaven.

As we age, we shrink in all the wrong places and the lips can be particularly affected. Not only do we lose the padded puckering bits, but the definition can get lost as well. So you don't look 'ducky', the goal with any lip treatment is to replace that lost tissue, not create a completely different mouth.

My goal with lip rejuvenation is simple: I want to restore definition so I don't look like I have nothing where my mouth should be! But beware: many people over-do this, and can lend up looking like a puffer fish in distress.

I also use PRP to help with collagen stimulation and to try and keep a semblance of moisture in my lips. I've had regular injections into the body of the lips as well as around them to prevent deeper lines forming. Some practitioners also use laser to stimulate tissue repair, although it seems that the jury is still out on this method's effectiveness (there's a concern that if you laser the lip lines then they'll disappear and the lip will lose shape).

As a general rule when it comes to reinstating lost tissue, the key is to build up the lost tissue over time. In the case of the lips, usually only a small amount of filler is required. If you push filler up into the area between your nose and lip line, it becomes very obvious that you have 'had some work done'. When you have had a treatment, people should say things like "you are looking fantastic and you don't need to get any work". If they notice the work you have done, it isn't being done right.

NANNA HANDS

In my mind, I've never had attractive hands. As I have aged I have been dismayed at the rapid degradation of the skin and tissue on the back of my hands. I feel as if I have gone from having 'normal' hands to the hands of one of those crones I read about in my childhood fairy stories! As we age, we lose tissue between the veins. If we are slim, those veins become quite prominent. Over the years I've tried various fillers to stimulate collagen growth and reinstate some of the original plumpness of my hands. I've also used PRP at times. The other thing that happens is the appearance of spots such as freckles and age spots. This is because hands are often exposed to the sun and even if you put sunscreen on, then this washes off leaving the skin exposed again. Despite religiously slathering sunscreen on my hand before leaving the house, I still have to fight the spots. My treatment protocol is below and I've found that it is the combination of approaches that gives the best results.

> **Filler.** This is the basic tool to help keep my hands from looking skeletal. Dr Kathy Gallagher treats my hands, and last time we used Volift® filler. It has worked really well, so I'll probably use it again next time.

> **Laser.** Used in conjunction with filler, this gives great results. Dr Bruce Williamson usually does my laser work and he uses a fractionated CO_2 laser to resurface the skin and to stimulate collagen growth. A word of caution, if you get your hands lasered, make sure you stagger the laser work up the arm so that is doesn't look like you have white gloves on; when the skin regrows it is lighter than the older skin on your arm.

> **PRP.** I've had this done intermittently. Bruce typically rubs it into any laser wounds and it seems to stimulate tissue regeneration to fast-track my recovery.

> **Cosmeceuticals.** I use a cosmeceutical as part of my regular skincare regime. Be sure your product includes active ingredients such as Vitamin C and retinol to promote skin rejuvenation. I am currently using products from Ultraceuticals.

NECK

As a child living in the country, I used to slather baby oil onto my face and neck an attempt to go brown. I'm a red haired (well, I was back then anyway!) freckled person and this was disastrous. I ended up with quite a discoloured neck as I aged.

The neck is one of those 'problem areas' that can really show our age. We all know and dread the 'turkey neck'. Let's not pretend, if we could avoid it we would! I live in hope that there will be a magic bullet and we will be delivered of what I think is one of the worst blights of ageing. I've tried many and varied treatments on the neck, including:

> **Erbium laser.** For treating staining due to sun damage and lack of care.

> **CO2 laser.** To improve skin texture.

> **PRP.** Used in conjunction with needling to improve collagen rejuvenation.

> **Ulthera and Ultraforma.** For tightening around my jaw line, neck and décolletage

> **Cosmeceuticals.** Used religiously, especially those containing Vitamin C, retinoid and sunscreen.

KATE'S SOLUTIONS

AREA	CONCERNS	TREATMENTS
Face	As soon as I become lean, I lose my facial fullness due to loss of fat pads above eyes leading to skeletal look. I've also got more wrinkles and lines which appear in odd places such as a crease line down one side of my face under my eye. I constantly combat spots and other signs of skin ageing.	Cosmeceuticals, fillers and volumisers, anti-wrinkle injections, CO2 laser treatments, stem cell injections and PRP injections. **Procedures:** ageslow.co/face-rejuvenation ageslow.co/wrinkle-injection ageslow.co/stem-cells ageslow.co/fat-harvesting
Lips	My lips have gradually lost tissue and become dryer and are in danger of going missing forever!	PRP, filler, Botox at the corners to prevent the inevitable down turn that accompanies ageing. **Procedure:** ageslow.co/lip-rejuvenation
Neck and chest	Sun damage, platysmal bands that stick out, increased skin laxity and getting 'turkey neck'.	Erbium laser, CO2 laser, PRP, Botox to relax the platysmal bands, Ultraformer ultrasound skin tightening, cosmeceuticals. **Procedure:** ageslow.co/neck-rejuvenation ageslow.co/prp-neck
Hands	I get lots of age spots as well as loss of tissue and fat so my veins pop out.	Filler, CO2 laser and PRP injections. **Procedure:** ageslow.co/hand-rejuvenation ageslow.co/prp-hand-rejuvenation
Skin laxity	Even though I'm fit, my skin has started to pull away from my muscle walls around my knees, under arms and event belly.	Ultraformer ultrasound skin tightening. **Procedure:** ageslow.co/skin-tightening
Spider veins	Am getting spider veins in my legs.	Sclerotherapy injections. **Procedure:** ageslow.co/vein-treatment

LESSONS I'VE LEARNED ON MY SKIN JOURNEY

> **Build up filler over time to reinstate shrunken areas.** Otherwise you'll look freakish rather than your normal self. We all know that 'plastic' look and it's not attractive.

> **Create an annual plan and find the right practitioner.** Interview to find one who is the best at the various treatments you want to do – there are many Jack-of-all-trades out there who are the master of none.

> **Embrace a multi-treatment approach.** It works best. A good example would be if you are going to do laser work, be sure to back up the skin rejuvenation effect with quality evidence-based cosmeceuticals.

> **Spread treatments out; do a little bit at a time.** A great example is the treatment of age spots. They seem to come in batches, so you need to regularly treat them.

> **Take the time to research details.** Remember that any investment that is long term is a strategic choice and not to be done in an ad hoc way. The more you know, the better you are equipped to make an informed decision.

> **Take manufacturer claims with a grain of salt.** It is often said in medical circles that 50 percent of what we think is the truth now will be proven to be incorrect in our lifetime. The question is, which 50 percent? I'm extremely wary when it comes to dogmatic people claiming to 'know' things to be completely, unalterably true. Often these people are not prepared to admit when they are wrong and that can present a danger to you as a patient.

> **Remember that sugar is the enemy of the skin.** It won't matter what else you do if you persist in bathing your cells in sugar, as sugar accelerates ageing. Do whatever it takes to reduce your sugar intake. I treat it as an addiction and have used hypnotherapy and other psychological methods to help me give it up.

> **Seek evidence-based treatments and the 'geeks' in love with them.** A case in point is the use of laser equipment. This treatment has given me great results, but it is not a risk-free area. The use of lasers is largely unregulated, so you need to be particularly cautious about practitioner claims. Lasers are a big investment and the practitioner's desire to pay it off can sometimes lead to inappropriate application.

> **Nitrous oxide can be your best friend on your cosmetic medicine journey.** Many practitioners downplay the pain involved with some treatments and it is easy to then feel disempowered if you are worried about it. The best practitioners recognise your concern around pain and are able to help you navigate your choices, meaning you aren't anxious and enjoy not only the results but also the treatment process itself.

> **Give things a go.** Don't start and stop and fiddle around, this will mean inconsistent results. If you are going to embark on a new skincare regime based on research and analysis of your needs, for instance, then stick to it and don't be swayed by the next fad you see advertised or that your friend recommends. The best results come from being consistent and deliberate with your choices. You need to set clear and measurable objectives so you know if you are achieving the results you desire.

INDEX